Best Practices

for Comprehensive Tobacco Control Programs

October 2007

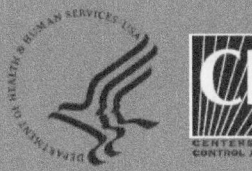

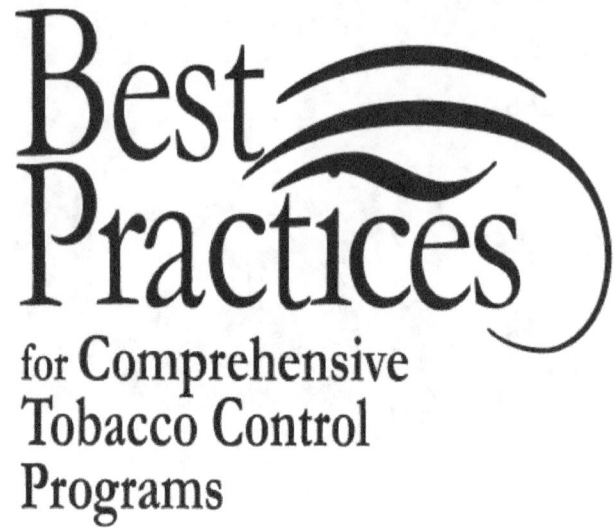

Best Practices

for Comprehensive Tobacco Control Programs

Suggested Citation

Centers for Disease Control and Prevention. *Best Practices for Comprehensive Tobacco Control Programs—2007*. Atlanta: U.S. Department of Health and Human Services, Centers for Disease Control and Prevention, National Center for Chronic Disease Prevention and Health Promotion, Office on Smoking and Health; October 2007. *Reprinted with corrections.*

Ordering Information

To download or order copies of this book,
go to www.cdc.gov/tobacco
or
to order single copies, call toll-free
1 (800) CDC-INFO
1 (800) 232-4636

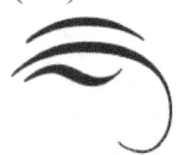

Best Practices for Comprehensive Tobacco Control Programs—2007

The following individuals from the Centers for Disease Control and Prevention,
Coordinating Center for Health Promotion, National Center for Chronic Disease Prevention
and Health Promotion, Office on Smoking and Health, were primary contributors
to the preparation of this publication:

Terry F. Pechacek, PhD, Associate Director for Science
Nicole A. Blair, MPH, Health Scientist
Corinne G. Husten, MD, MPH, Chief, Epidemiology Branch
Peter Mariolis, PhD, Health Scientist
Gabrielle B. Starr, MA, Health Scientist

Valuable input was provided by an expert panel,
whose members are identified in Appendix A.

Additional contributions were provided by:

Jan Stone–*American Cancer Society*; Donna Vallone, PhD, MPH–*American Legacy Foundation*;
Patricia Tarango–*Arizona Department of Health Services*; Lori Asbury–*Frankel, an Arc Worldwide Company*;
David W. Cowling, PhD, Colleen Stevens, MSW–*California Department of Public Health*; Danny McGoldrick,
Meg Gallogly, MPH–*Campaign for Tobacco-free Kids*; Karen DeLeeuw, MSW–*Colorado Department
of Public Health and Environment*; Tim McAfee, MD, MPH, Mary Kate Salley, BA–*Free and Clear*;
Donna Warner, MA, MBA–*Massachusetts Department of Health*; Ursula Bauer, PhD, MPH–*New York
State Department of Health*; Linda Bailey, JD, MHS–*North American Quitline Consortium*; Joe Gitchell–
PinneyAssociates; Todd Rogers, PhD–*Public Health Institute*; Matthew C. Farrelly, PhD, Brett R. Loomis, MS,
Kristin Thomas, MSPH–*RTI International*; Douglas Luke, PhD, Nancy Mueller, MPH–*Saint Louis University*

Mahshid V. Amini; Gloria Bryan, PhD, RN; Ralph Caraballo, PhD; Galen Cole, PhD, MPH; Kevin T. Collins,
MPA; Steve DePaul; Monica H. Eischen, BS; Martha Engstrom, MS; Erik M. Friedly; Lynn Hughley, BS;
Paul Hunting, MPH; Natasha Jamison, MPH; Jerelyn Jordan, BA; Rachel Kaufmann, MPH, PhD; Nicole
Kuiper, MPH; Brick Lancaster, MA, CHES; Joel London, MPH; Ann Malarcher, PhD; Robert K. Merritt, MA;
Cynthia Mitchell; Elizabeth Mitchell, PhD; Rebecca Murphy, PhD; Barbara Z. Park, RDH, MPH;
Linda Pederson, PhD; Gabrielle Promoff, MA; Jennifer H. Reynolds, MPH; Brenda A. Richards, RN, MHS;
Maria Rivera-Trudeau, MBA; Abby Rosenthal, MPH; Patti R. Seikus, MPH; Dana Shelton, MPH;
Karen Siener, MPH; Monica Swann, MBA; Debra S. Torres, MPH–*CDC, Office on Smoking and Health*

Lisa C. Barrios, DrPH; Rebekah Buckley, MPH, CRT, AE-C; John Canfield, MEd, CHES; Linda Crossett,
RDH; Laura Kahn, PhD; Adriane King, MPH; William Potts-Datema, MS–*CDC, Division
of Adolescent and School Health*

Patricia A. Stephens, PhD; Faye L. Wong, MPH–*CDC, National Center for Chronic Disease
Prevention and Health Promotion*

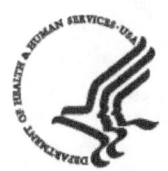

U.S. Department of Health and Human Services
Centers for Disease Control and Prevention
National Center for Chronic Disease Prevention and Health Promotion
Office on Smoking and Health

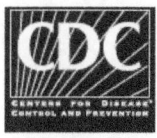

Table of Contents

Best Practices for Comprehensive Tobacco Control Programs

Tobacco* use is the single most preventable cause of death and disease in the United States. People begin using tobacco in early adolescence; almost all first use occurs before age 18. An estimated 45 million American adults currently smoke cigarettes. Annually, cigarette smoking causes approximately 438,000 deaths. For every person who dies from tobacco use, another 20 suffer with at least one serious tobacco-related illness. Half of all long-term smokers die prematurely from smoking-related causes. In 2004, this addiction costs the nation more than $96 billion per year in direct medical expenses as well as more than $97 billion annually in lost productivity. Furthermore, exposure to secondhand smoke causes premature death and disease in nonsmokers. In 2005, the Society of Actuaries estimated that the effects of exposure to secondhand smoke cost the United States $10 billion per year.

Nearly 50 years have elapsed since the first Surgeon General's Advisory Committee concluded: "Cigarette smoking is a health hazard of sufficient importance in the United States to warrant appropriate remedial action." There now is a robust evidence base about effective interventions. Yet, despite this progress, the United States has not yet achieved the goal of making tobacco use a rare behavior. A 2007 Institute of Medicine (IOM) report presented a blueprint for action to "reduce smoking so substantially that it is no longer a public health problem for our nation." The two-pronged strategy for achieving this goal includes not only strengthening and fully implementing currently proven tobacco control measures, but also changing the regulatory landscape to permit policy innovations. Foremost among the IOM recommendations is that each state should fund a comprehensive tobacco control program at the level recommended by the Centers for Disease Control and Prevention (CDC).

We know how to end the epidemic. Evidence-based, statewide tobacco control programs that are comprehensive, sustained, and accountable have been shown to reduce smoking rates, tobacco-related deaths, and diseases caused by smoking. Recommendations that define a comprehensive statewide tobacco control intervention have been provided in the Surgeon General's reports *Reducing Tobacco Use* (2000) and *The Health Consequences of Involuntary Exposure to Tobacco Smoke* (2006),

the Task Force for Community Preventive Services' *Guide to Community Preventive Services* (2005), IOM's *Ending the Tobacco Problem: A Blueprint for the Nation* (2007), the Public Health Service's Clinical Practice Guideline *Treating Tobacco Use and Dependence* (2000), and the National Institutes of Health's State-of-the-Science Conference Statement *Tobacco Use: Prevention, Cessation, and Control* (2006) and President's Cancer Panel Annual Report *Promoting Health Lifestyles: Policy, Program and Personal Recommendations for Reducing Cancer Risk* (2007).

A comprehensive statewide tobacco control program is a coordinated effort to establish smoke-free policies and social norms, to promote and assist tobacco users to quit, and to prevent initiation of tobacco use. This comprehensive approach combines educational, clinical, regulatory, economic, and social strategies. Research has documented the effectiveness of laws and policies in a comprehensive tobacco control effort to protect the public from secondhand smoke exposure, promote cessation, and prevent initiation, including increasing the unit price of tobacco products and implementing smoking bans through policies, regulations, and laws; providing insurance coverage of tobacco use treatment; and limiting minors' access to tobacco products. Additionally, research has shown greater effectiveness with multi-component intervention efforts that integrate the implementation of programmatic and policy interventions to influence social norms, systems, and networks.

---

* In this document, the term "tobacco" refers to the use of manufactured, commercial tobacco products including, but not limited to, cigarettes, smokeless tobacco, and cigars.

Executive Summary

This document updates *Best Practices for Comprehensive Tobacco Control Programs—August 1999.* This updated edition describes an integrated programmatic structure for implementing interventions proven to be effective and provides the recommended level of state investment to reach these goals and reduce tobacco use in each state. It is important to recognize that these individual components must work together to produce the synergistic effects of a comprehensive tobacco control program. Based on the evidence of effectiveness documented in scientific literature, the most effective population-based approaches have been defined within the following overarching components:

I. State and Community Interventions

State and community interventions include supporting and implementing programs and policies to influence societal organizations, systems, and networks that encourage and support individuals to make behavior choices consistent with tobacco-free norms. The social norm change model presumes that durable change occurs through shifts in the social environment, initially or ultimately, at the grassroots level across local communities. State and community interventions unite a range of integrated programmatic activities, including local and statewide policies and programs, chronic disease and tobacco-related disparity elimination initiatives, and interventions specifically aimed at influencing youth.

II. Health Communication Interventions

An effective state health communication intervention should deliver strategic, culturally appropriate, and high-impact messages in sustained and adequately funded campaigns integrated into the overall state tobacco program effort. Traditional health communication interventions and counter-marketing strategies employ a wide range of efforts, including paid television, radio, billboard, print, and web-based advertising at the state and local levels; media advocacy through public relations efforts, such as press releases, local events, media literacy, and health promotion activities; and efforts to reduce or replace tobacco industry sponsorship and promotions. Innovations in health communication interventions include more focused targeting of specific audiences as well as fostering message development and distribution by the target audience through appropriate channels.

III. Cessation Interventions

Interventions to increase cessation encompass a broad array of policy, system, and population-based measures. System-based initiatives should ensure that all patients seen in the health care system are screened for tobacco use, receive brief interventions to help them quit, and are offered more intensive counseling services and FDA-approved cessation medications. Cessation quitlines are effective and have the potential to reach large numbers of tobacco users. Quitlines also serve as a resource for busy health care providers, who provide the brief intervention and discuss medication options and then link tobacco users to quitline cessation services for more intensive counseling. Optimally, quitline counseling should be made available to all tobacco users willing to access the service.

IV. Surveillance and Evaluation

State surveillance is the process of monitoring tobacco-related attitudes, behaviors, and health outcomes at regular intervals. Statewide surveillance should monitor the achievement of overall program goals. Program evaluation is used to assess the implementation and outcomes of a program, increase efficiency and impact over time, and demonstrate accountability. A comprehensive state tobacco control plan—with well-defined goals; objectives; and short-term, intermediate, and long-term indicators—requires appropriate surveillance and evaluation data systems. Collecting baseline data related to each objective and performance indicator is critical to ensuring that program-related effects can be clearly measured. For this reason, surveillance and evaluation systems must have first priority in the planning process.

V. Administration and Management

Effective tobacco prevention and control programs require substantial funding to implement, thus making critical the need for sound fiscal management. Internal capacity within a state health department is essential for program sustainability, efficacy, and efficiency. Sufficient capacity enables programs to plan their strategic efforts, provide strong leadership, and foster collaboration between the state and local tobacco control communities. An adequate number of skilled staff is also necessary to provide or facilitate program oversight, technical assistance, and training.

The primary objective of the recommended statewide comprehensive tobacco control program is to reduce the personal and societal burden of tobacco-related deaths and illnesses. Research shows that the more states spend on comprehensive tobacco control programs, the greater the reductions in smoking—and the longer states invest in such programs, the greater and faster the impact. States that invest more fully in comprehensive tobacco control programs have seen cigarette sales drop more than twice as much as in the United States as a whole, and smoking prevalence among adults and youth has declined faster as spending for tobacco control programs has increased.

In California, home of the longest-running comprehensive tobacco control program, adult smoking rates declined from 22.7% in 1988 to 13.3% in 2006. As a result, compared with the rest of the country, heart disease deaths and lung cancer incidence in California have declined at accelerated rates. Due to the program-related reductions in smoking, lung cancer incidence has been declining four times faster in that state than in the rest of the nation. Among women in California, the rate of lung cancer deaths decreased while it increased in other parts of the country. Because of this accelerated decline, California has the potential to be the first state in which lung cancer is no longer the leading cancer cause of death.

Implementing a comprehensive tobacco control program structure at the CDC-recommended levels of investment would have a substantial impact. For example, if each state sustained its recommended level of funding for 5 years, an estimated 5 million fewer people in this country would smoke. As a result, hundreds of thousands of premature tobacco-related deaths would be prevented. Longer-term investments would have even greater effects.

The tobacco use epidemic can be stopped. We know what works, and if we were to fully implement the proven strategies, we could prevent the staggering toll that tobacco takes on our families and in our communities. We could accelerate the declines in cardiovascular mortality, reduce chronic obstructive pulmonary disease, and once again make lung cancer a rare disease. If we as a nation fully protected our children from secondhand smoke, more than one million asthma attacks and lung and ear infections in children could be prevented. With sustained implementation of state tobacco control programs and policies (e.g., increases in the unit price of tobacco products), IOM's best-case scenario of reducing adult tobacco prevalence to 10% by 2025 would be attainable.

Tobacco use is the single most preventable cause of death and disease in the United States. An estimated 45 million American adults currently smoke cigarettes.[1] Smoking harms nearly every organ in the body and half of all long-term smokers die prematurely from smoking-related disease.[2] All tobacco products, including smokeless tobacco and cigars, cause cancer, and all forms of tobacco are addictive.[3,4] Secondhand smoke causes premature death and disease in children and adults who do not smoke.[5] There is no risk-free level of exposure to secondhand smoke.[5]

Most people begin using tobacco as adolescents. Although rates of youth smoking increased dramatically in the early 1990s, after increased implementation of evidence-based interventions, youth smoking declined 40% from 1997 to 2003. Unfortunately, recent data indicate this decline appears to have stalled.[6] Several factors may have contributed to this lack of continued decline. These factors include smaller annual increases in the retail price of cigarettes during 2003–2005 compared with 1997–2003, decreased exposure among youth to effective mass media smoking-prevention campaigns, less funding for comprehensive statewide tobacco-use prevention programs, and substantial increases in tobacco industry expenditures on tobacco advertising and promotion in the United States.[6] If current patterns of smoking persist in this country, more than six million youth will die more than 10 years prematurely due to smoking.[7]

In 1964 the Surgeon General's Advisory Committee concluded: "Cigarette smoking is a health hazard of sufficient importance in the United States to warrant appropriate remedial action."[8] Yet, since 1964, more than 12 million tobacco-related deaths have occurred in the United States.[2] Each year in this country, there are approximately 438,000 additional premature deaths from tobacco-related diseases.[9] Also, for every person who dies from tobacco use, 20 others currently suffer with at least one serious tobacco-related illness.[10]

In 2007, the Institute of Medicine (IOM) released *Ending the Tobacco Problem: A Blueprint for the Nation,* with the goal of reducing smoking "so substantially that it is no longer a significant public health problem for our nation."[11] The IOM Committee on Reducing Tobacco Use concluded that this ultimate goal could be achieved with a two-pronged strategy: strengthening and fully implementing traditional tobacco control measures, and changing the regulatory landscape to permit policy innovations.[11] The IOM Committee concluded that there was compelling evidence that comprehensive state tobacco programs could achieve substantial reductions in tobacco use, and that to effectively reduce tobacco use, "states must maintain over time a comprehensive integrated tobacco control strategy."[11] On the basis of this evidence, the lead recommendation in the IOM report stated:

> **Each state should fund state tobacco control activities at the level recommended by the CDC. A reasonable target for each state is in the range of $15 to $20 per capita, depending on the state's population, demography, and prevalence of tobacco use.[11]**

If, starting in fiscal year 2009, all states were to fully fund their tobacco control programs at the updated CDC-recommended level of investment described in this report, in 5 years, an estimated 5 million fewer people in this country would smoke, and hundreds of thousands of premature tobacco-related deaths would be prevented each year. Longer investments will have even greater effects. With fully funded and sustained state tobacco control programs and policies (e.g., increases in the unit price of tobacco products), IOM's best-case scenario of reducing tobacco prevalence to 10% by 2025 would be attainable.

States that have made larger investments in comprehensive tobacco control programs have seen cigarette sales drop more than twice as much as in the United States as a whole, and smoking prevalence among adults and youth has declined faster as spending for tobacco control programs increased.[12-14] In Florida, between 1998 and 2002, a comprehensive prevention program anchored by an aggressive youth-oriented health communications campaign, reduced smoking rates among middle school students by 50% and among high school students by 35%.[15] Other

Introduction

states, such as Maine, New York, and Washington, have seen 45% to 60% reductions in youth smoking rates with sustained comprehensive statewide programs.[16-18] Between 2000 and 2006, the New York State Tobacco Control Program reported that the prevalence of both adult and youth smoking declined faster in New York than in the United States as a whole.[18] Adult smoking prevalence declined 16% and smoking among high school students declined by 40%, resulting in more than 600,000 fewer smokers in the state over the 7-year intervention period.[18]

According to the American Cancer Society (ACS), even by the most conservative estimates, more than 40% of the reduction in male cancer deaths between 1991 and 2003 was due to the declines in smoking over the last half of the 20th century.[19] Before cigarette smoking became common, lung cancer was a rare disease. Now lung cancer is the leading cancer cause of death for both men and women, killing an estimated 160,000 people in this country each year.[20] ACS estimates that approximately 87% of these deaths are caused by smoking and exposure to secondhand smoke.[19] Additionally, more than 100,000 deaths from lung diseases, and more than 140,000 premature deaths from heart disease and stroke are caused each year by smoking and exposure to secondhand smoke.[2]

Research shows that the more states spend on sustained comprehensive tobacco control programs, the greater the reductions in smoking—and the longer states invest in such programs, the greater and faster the impact.[12] In California, home of the longest-running comprehensive program, smoking rates among adults declined from 22.7% in 1988 to 13.3% in 2006.[21] As a result, compared with the rest of the country, heart disease deaths and lung cancer incidence in California have declined at accelerated rates. Among women in California, the rate of lung cancer deaths decreased while it continued to increase in other parts of the country.[22] Overall, from 1987–1998, approximately 11,000 cases of lung cancer were avoided.[23] Since 1998, lung cancer incidence in California has been declining four times faster than in the rest of the nation.[22,24]

Because of this accelerated decline, California has the potential to be the first state in which lung cancer is no longer the leading cancer cause of death. Unfortunately, at the present time, this projection cannot be made for the rest of the nation.

Comprehensive Tobacco Control Programs

The mission of comprehensive tobacco control programs is to reduce disease, disability, and death related to tobacco use. A comprehensive approach—one that optimizes synergy from applying a mix of educational, clinical, regulatory, economic, and social strategies—has been established as the guiding principle for eliminating the health and economic burden of tobacco use.[25]

The goals for comprehensive tobacco control programs include:
- Preventing initiation among youth and young adults
- Promoting quitting among adults and youth
- Eliminating exposure to secondhand smoke
- Identifying and eliminating tobacco-related disparities among population groups

CDC has prepared these "best practices" to help states organize their tobacco control program efforts into an integrated and effective structure that uses and maximizes interventions proven to be effective and to operate at the scale that would be required to ultimately eliminate the burden of tobacco use. In *Best Practices for Comprehensive Tobacco Control Programs—August 1999,* recommendations were based on the extant scientific literature and the experience of large-scale, sustained state programs in California and Massachusetts.[26] After *Best Practices* was published in 1999, overall funding for state tobacco control programs more than doubled. States restructured their tobacco control programs to align with CDC's goals and programmatic recommendations. Eight states—Arizona, Arkansas, Colorado, Delaware, Indiana, Massachusetts, Minnesota, and Mississippi—have met CDC's minimum funding recommendation for one or more years; Maine has met the minimum funding recommendation every year. In fiscal year 2007, three states—Colorado, Delaware, and Maine—met the minimum recommended level of funding. With this growth in state capacity and a focus on proven interventions, evidence demonstrating the effectiveness of comprehensive programs has steadily increased. *Best Practices for Comprehensive Tobacco Control Programs—2007* has utilized this robust evidence base to update the recommendations.

National Initiatives

A comprehensive approach to tobacco prevention and control requires coordination and collaboration across the federal government, across the nation, and within each state. The federal government has undertaken a number of important activities that provide a foundation for state action. Scientific data about the extent of tobacco use, its impact, and effective interventions to reduce its use have been generated and disseminated by several federal agencies, including CDC, the National Institutes of Health (NIH), the Substance Abuse and Mental Health Services Administration (SAMHSA), and the Agency for Healthcare Research and Quality.

NIH's National Cancer Institute (NCI) has supported innovative intervention studies, including mass media and school trials and large-scale demonstration projects such as the American Stop Smoking Intervention Study for Cancer Prevention (ASSIST) and Community Intervention Trial for Smoking Cessation (COMMIT).[25,27-29] CDC also provided state support through the Initiatives to Mobilize for the Prevention and Control of Tobacco Use (IMPACT) program.[25] In 1999, the National Tobacco Control Program (NTCP) was launched, combining NCI and CDC initiatives into one coordinated national program funded and managed by CDC. NTCP provides technical assistance and limited funding to all 50 states, the District of Columbia, and seven territories, as well as Tribal Support Centers and National Networks of specific populations. CDC funding is designed to support and leverage state funding for evidence-based interventions and to help states evaluate their program efforts. The National Network of Tobacco Cessation Quitlines was developed through a partnership among CDC, the NCI Cancer Information Service, the North American Quitline Consortium, and the states. This system provides callers from across the nation with a single, toll-free access point (1-800-QUIT NOW) that automatically routes them to their state's telephone-based cessation services. Additionally, SAMHSA

implements the Synar regulation to reduce youth access to tobacco products through state-level retail compliance activities.

The federal government has also supported a number of national and state tobacco use surveys among adults and youth through the CDC (Behavioral Risk Factor Surveillance System, National Health Interview Survey, Youth Risk Behavior Surveillance System, national and state Adult Tobacco Surveys, and national and state Youth Tobacco Surveys), NIH (Current Population Survey Tobacco Use Supplement and Monitoring the Future Study), and SAMHSA (National Survey on Drug Use and Health). These surveys provide complementary data obtained from various populations that are useful and important for monitoring and evaluating progress in tobacco control.

National partners also play a critical role in tobacco prevention and control efforts. For example, the American Legacy Foundation's social marketing campaign, truth®, began in early 2000. It reinforces state-based youth prevention efforts and has been independently associated with substantial declines in youth smoking.[30] Americans for Nonsmokers' Rights provides extensive technical assistance and guidance to states and municipalities as they engage in the process of passing and implementing smoke-free indoor air policies as well as exposing tobacco industry strategies that can undermine smoke-free initiatives. The Robert Wood Johnson Foundation has supported research to document the effectiveness of policies and programs and helped to build the advocacy and communications infrastructure to advance those policies to reduce smoking and help people lead healthier lives. The American Cancer Society, American Heart Association, and American Lung Association provide strong national, state, and local advocacy leadership on tobacco control policy issues, as well as community support through local offices around the country. The Tobacco Control Legal Consortium, a network of legal programs supporting tobacco control policy change, works to assist communities and increase legal resources available for tobacco control. The Tobacco Technical Assistance Consortium supports the effectiveness of tobacco control programs by providing technical assistance and training to state and local programs, partners, and coalitions. The Campaign for Tobacco-

Introduction

programs, and provides technical assistance for policy interventions. The Association of State and Territorial Health Officials, the National Association of County and City Health Officials, and the National Association of Local Boards of Health provide state and local health officials with information and resources, including *Joint Policy Action Steps Toward Tobacco Use Prevention and Control,* which support the development and maintenance of strong state and local tobacco control policies and programs to achieve the *Healthy People 2010* tobacco use-related health objectives for the nation.[31,32]

Although a number of critical activities to curb tobacco use occur at the national level, state and local community action is essential to ensure the success of tobacco control interventions. Almost 90% of funds for tobacco control interventions come from the states through tobacco excise tax revenues and tobacco settlement payments. Furthermore, it is the policies, partnerships, and intervention activities that occur at the state and local levels that ultimately lead to social norm and behavior change. In acknowledging the essential and unique roles that states and communities play in tobacco control efforts, these best practices provide technical information and evidence-based benchmarks to assist states in designing comprehensive programs. Communities, in turn, support comprehensive programs by implementing evidence-based initiatives at the local level. For example, although the quitline portal number and structure of the National Network of Tobacco Cessation Quitlines were established through partnerships at the national level, states provide the foundation for this system by maintaining their quitline services and promoting their use through broadcast media. Communities can further promote this service through local channels, such as hospitals, health care systems, local newspapers, and community and civic organizations.

Implementing Best Practices for Comprehensive Tobacco Control Programs

This document draws upon best practices determined by evidence-based analyses of scientific literature and outcomes of comprehensive state tobacco control programs and interventions. CDC recommends that states implement evidence-based tobacco control programs that are comprehensive, sustainable, and accountable. This guidance document describes an integrated budget structure for implementing interventions proven to be effective and the recommended state investment that would be required to reduce, and ultimately eliminate, tobacco use in each state.

Best Practices for Comprehensive Tobacco Control Programs—2007 refines the guidance provided in 1999, reflecting additional state experiences in implementing comprehensive programs and new scientific literature since its original release.[33] A 2002–2003 evaluation of 10 states' implementation of *Best Practices—1999* found that the document provided an effective framework for tobacco control programs, but the number of categories was somewhat cumbersome to implement and convey to decision makers.[34]

In December 2006, technical consultation was sought from a panel of experts regarding the best available evidence to determine updated cost parameters and the metrics to calculate them for major components of a comprehensive tobacco control program. The panel generally agreed that although the types of interventions and funding formulas remained sound, funding estimates would be expected to increase to account for changes in state population and inflation since the 1999 publication. The panel also generally agreed that although none of the components should be eliminated, the framework should be consolidated into five categories to reflect the need for integrated approaches and the actual practices of state programs. A listing of participants in the expert panel is provided in Appendix A.

As a result of evidence-based analysis of tobacco excise tax-funded and tobacco settlement-funded programs, in-depth involvement with all 50 state tobacco control programs and the District of Columbia, and published evidence of effective tobacco control strategies, CDC recommends that states establish and sustain tobacco control programs that contain the following overarching components:

- State and Community Interventions
- Health Communication Interventions
- Cessation Interventions
- Surveillance and Evaluation
- Administration and Management

Information for each of these funding categories includes

- Justification for the program intervention
- Budget recommendations for successful implementation
- Core resources to assist implementation
- References to scientific literature

As with the funding guidance first published in 1999, recommended annual costs can vary within the lower and upper estimate provided for each state. Therefore, to better assist states, specific guidance is now provided regarding each state's recommended level of investment within their range. These recommended levels of annual investment factor in state-specific variables, such as the overall population; the prevalence of tobacco use; the proportion of the population that is uninsured, receiving publicly financed insurance, or living at or near the poverty level; infrastructure costs; the number of local health units; geographic size; the targeted reach for quitline services; and the cost and complexity of conducting mass media to reach targeted audiences, such as youth, racial/ethnic minorities, tobacco users interested in quitting, or people of low socioeconomic status. The 1999 funding formulas and 2007 adjustments are provided in Appendix B.

On the basis of these different factors, the annual investment needed to implement the recommended program components has been estimated to range from $9.23 to $18.02 per capita across 50 states and the District of Columbia. Among some states—particularly those with smaller populations, lower smoking prevalence, and inexpensive media markets without much state crossover—these recommended levels of investment are quite similar to the 1999 lower estimate adjusted for inflation. However, states with greater numbers of tobacco users, media markets that also include major metropolitan areas from neighboring states, or large and diverse populations may find recommended funding levels that are at the higher end of the funding range for some or all of the program components.

While each state's analysis of their priorities should shape decisions about funding allocations for each recommended program component, it remains clear that greater investments in comprehensive statewide programs lead to faster and larger declines in smoking rates and in smoking-related disease and death.[12-14]

Best Practices for Comprehensive Tobacco Control Programs—2007 provides evidence to support each of the five components of a comprehensive program. However, besides acknowledging the importance of the individual program components, it is equally important to recognize why these individual components must work together to produce the synergistic effects of a comprehensive program. A comprehensive approach, with the combination and coordination of all five program components, has shown to be most effective at preventing tobacco use initiation and promoting cessation.[33,35,36]

Each day in the United States—
- The tobacco industry spends nearly $36 million to market and promote its products.[37]
- Almost 4,000 adolescents start smoking.[38]
- Approximately 1,200 current and former smokers die prematurely from tobacco-related diseases.[9]
- The nation spends more than $260 million in direct medical costs related to smoking.[7]
- The nation experiences nearly $270 million in lost productivity due to premature deaths from tobacco-related diseases.[7]

The tobacco use epidemic can be stopped. We know what works, and if we were to fully implement the proven strategies, we could prevent the staggering toll that tobacco takes on our families and communities. We could accelerate the declines in cardiovascular mortality, reduce chronic obstructive pulmonary disease, and once again make lung cancer a rare disease. If we fully protected our children from secondhand smoke, more than a million asthma attacks and lung and ear infections in children could be prevented.[5,39]

Investing in and implementing what we know works will end the tobacco use epidemic.

Introduction

General Planning Resources

Institute of Medicine. *Ending the Tobacco Problem: A Blueprint for the Nation.* Washington, DC: National Academies Press; 2007.

Zaza S, Briss PA, Harris KW editors. *The Guide to Community Preventive Services: What Works to Promote Health?* New York: Oxford University Press; 2005. Available at http://www.thecommunityguide.org/tobacco/default htm.

California Department of Health Services. *A Model for Change: The California Experience in Tobacco Control.* Sacramento: California Department of Health Services; 1998. Available at http://www.dhs.ca.gov/tobacco/documents/pubs/modelforchange.pdf.

U.S. Department of Health and Human Services. *Reducing Tobacco Use: A Report of the Surgeon General.* Atlanta: U.S. Department of Health and Human Services, Centers for Disease Control and Prevention, National Center for Chronic Disease Prevention and Health Promotion, Office on Smoking and Health; 2000. Available at http://www.cdc.gov/tobacco/data_statistics/sgr/sgr_2000/index htm.

National Cancer Institute. *Community-Based Interventions for Smokers: The COMMIT Field Experience.* Tobacco Control Monograph No. 6. Bethesda, MD: National Institutes of Health; 1995. NIH Pub. No. 95-4028. Available at http://cancercontrol.cancer.gov/tcrb/monographs/6/index.html.

National Cancer Institute. *ASSIST: Shaping the Future of Tobacco Prevention and Control.* Tobacco Control Monograph No. 16. Bethesda, MD: National Institutes of Health; 2005. NIH Pub No.05-5645. Available at http://cancercontrol.cancer.gov/tcrb/monographs/16/index html.

National Cancer Institute. *Evaluating ASSIST: A Blueprint for Understanding State-level Tobacco Control.* Tobacco Control Monograph No. 17. Bethesda, MD: National Institutes of Health; 2006. NIH Pub. No. 06-6058. Available at http://cancercontrol.cancer.gov/tcrb/monographs/17/index.html.

National Cancer Institute. *Greater Than the Sum: Systems Thinking in Tobacco Control.* Tobacco Control Monograph No. 18. Bethesda, MD: National Institutes of Health; 2007. NIH Pub No.06-6085. Available at http://cancercontrol.cancer.gov/tcrb/monographs/18/index html.

National Association of County and City Health Officials, National Association of Local Boards of Health, and Association of State and Territorial Health Officials. *Joint Policy Action Steps Toward Tobacco Use Prevention and Control.* Washington, DC: National Association of County and City Health Officials; 2007. Available at http://www naccho.org/topics/HPDP/documents/FINALJPAS7-07.pdf.

U.S. Department of Health and Human Services. *Healthy People 2010. Volume 2.* Washington, DC: U.S. Government Printing Office; 2000. Available at http://www healthypeople.gov/Document/HTML/Volume2/27Tobacco.htm.

Centers for Disease Control and Prevention. Smoking & Tobacco Use website. Available at www.cdc.gov/tobacco.

Centers for Disease Control and Prevention. State Tobacco Activities Tracking and Evaluation (STATE) System. Available at http://www nccd.cdc.gov/tobacco/STATEsystem.

References

1. Centers for Disease Control and Prevention. Tobacco use among adults—United States, 2005. *MMWR* 2006;55(42):1145–1148.
2. U.S. Department of Health and Human Services. *The Health Consequences of Smoking: A Report of the Surgeon General.* Atlanta: U.S. Department of Health and Human Services, Centers for Disease Control and Prevention, National Center for Chronic Disease Prevention and Health Promotion, Office on Smoking and Health; 2004.
3. Institute of Medicine. *Clearing the Smoke: Assessing the Science Base for Tobacco Harm Reduction.* Washington, DC: National Academies Press; 2001.
4. U.S. Department of Health and Human Services. *The Health Consequences of Smoking: Nicotine Addiction. A Report of the Surgeon General.* Rockville, MD: U.S. Department of Health and Human Services, Public Health Service, Centers for Disease Control, Center for Health Promotion and Education, Office on Smoking and Health; 1988.
5. U.S. Department of Health and Human Services. *The Health Consequences of Involuntary Exposure to Tobacco Smoke: A Report of the Surgeon General.* Atlanta: U.S. Department of Health and Human Services, Centers for Disease Control and Prevention, Coordinating Center for Health Promotion, National Center for Chronic Disease Prevention and Health Promotion, Office on Smoking and Health; 2006.
6. Centers for Disease Control and Prevention. Cigarette use among high school students—United States, 1991–2005. *MMWR* 2006;55(26):724–726.
7. Centers for Disease Control and Prevention. *Sustaining State Programs for Tobacco Control: Data Highlights 2006.* Atlanta: U.S. Department of Health and Human Services, Centers for Disease Control and Prevention, National Center for Chronic Disease Prevention and Health Promotion, Office on Smoking and Health; 2006.
8. U.S. Department of Health, Education, and Welfare. *Smoking and Health: Report of the Advisory Committee to the Surgeon General of the Public Health Service.* Washington, DC: U.S. Department of Health, Education, and Welfare, Public Health Service, Center for Disease Control; 1964. PHS Publication No. 1103.
9. Centers for Disease Control and Prevention. Annual smoking-attributable mortality, years of potential life lost, and productivity losses—United States, 1997-2001. *MMWR* 2005;54(25):625–628.
10. Centers for Disease Control and Prevention. Cigarette smoking-attributable morbidity—United States, 2000. *MMWR* 2003;52(35):842–844.
11. Institute of Medicine. *Ending the Tobacco Problem: A Blueprint for the Nation.* Washington, DC: National Academies Press; 2007.
12. Farrelly MC, Pechacek TP, Chaloupka FJ. The impact of tobacco control program expenditures on aggregate cigarette sales: 1981-2000. *Journal of Health Economics* 2003;22(5):843–859.
13. Tauras JA, Chaloupka FJ, Farrelly MC, Giovino GA, Wakefield M, Johnston LD, et al. State tobacco control spending and youth smoking. *American Journal of Public Health* 2005;954(2):338–344.
14. Farrelly MC, Pechacek TF, Thomas KY, Nelson D. The impact of tobacco control programs on adult smoking. *American Journal of Public Health.* In press.
15. Bauer UE, Johnson TM, Hopkins RS, Brooks RG. Changes in youth cigarette use and intentions following implementation of a tobacco control program. *JAMA* 2000;284(6):723–728.
16. Centers for Disease Control and Prevention. Youth Risk Behavior Surveillance System, Youth Online Comprehensive Results. Available at http://apps.nccd.cdc.gov/yrbss/.
17. Washington State Department of Health. *Tobacco Prevention & Control Program Progress Report, March 2007: Producing Results for a Healthier Washington.* Olympia, WA: Washington State Department of Health; 2007.
18. RTI International. *Fourth Annual Independent Evaluation Report of New York's Tobacco Control Program.* Albany, NY: New York State Department of Health; 2007.
19. American Cancer Society. *Cancer Prevention & Early Detection Facts & Figures 2007.* Atlanta: American Cancer Society; 2007.
20. American Cancer Society. *Cancer Facts & Figures 2007.* Atlanta: American Cancer Society; 2007.
21. California Department of Health Services. New data show 91 percent of California women don't smoke. News Release No. 07-37. May 22, 2007. Available at http://www.dhs.ca.gov/tobacco/documents/press/2007Releaseof2006PrevData.pdf.
22. Centers for Disease Control and Prevention. Declines in lung cancer rates—California, 1988–1997. *MMWR* 2000;49(47):1066–1069.
23. Barnoya J, Glantz S. Association of the California tobacco control program with declines in lung cancer incidence. *Cancer Causes and Control,* 2004;15(7):689-695.

Introduction

24. California Department of Health Services. *California Tobacco Control Update 2006: The Social Norm Change Approach*. Sacramento: California Department of Health Services; 2006.

25. U.S. Department of Health and Human Services. *Reducing Tobacco Use: A Report of the Surgeon General*. Atlanta: U.S. Department of Health and Human Services, Centers for Disease Control and Prevention, National Center for Chronic Disease Prevention and Health Promotion, Office on Smoking and Health; 2000.

26. Centers for Disease Control and Prevention. *Best Practices for Comprehensive Tobacco Control Programs—August 1999*. Atlanta: U.S. Department of Health and Human Services; 1999.

27. National Cancer Institute. *Community-Based Interventions for Smokers: The COMMIT Field Experience*. Tobacco Control Monograph No. 6. Bethesda, MD: National Institutes of Health; 1995. NIH Pub. No. 95-4028.

28. National Cancer Institute. *ASSIST: Shaping the Future of Tobacco Prevention and Control*. Tobacco Control Monograph No. 16. Bethesda, MD: National Institutes of Health; 2005. NIH Pub No.05-5645.

29. National Cancer Institute. *Evaluating ASSIST: A Blueprint for Understanding State-level Tobacco Control*. Tobacco Control Monograph No. 17. Bethesda, MD: National Institutes of Health; 2006. NIH Pub. No. 06-6058.

30. Farrelly MC, Davis KC, Haviland L, Messeri P, Healton CG. Evidence of a dose-response relationship between "truth" antismoking ads and youth smoking prevalence. *American Journal of Public Health* 2005;95(3):425–431.

31. National Association of County and City Health Officials, National Association of Local Boards of Health, and Association of State and Territorial Health Officials. *Joint Policy Action Steps Toward Tobacco Use Prevention and Control*. Washington, DC: National Association of County and City Health Officials; 2007.

32. U.S. Department of Health and Human Services. *Healthy People 2010. Volume 2*. Washington, DC: U.S. Government Printing Office; 2000.

33. Zaza S, Briss PA, Harris KW, editors. *The Guide to Community Preventive Services: What Works to Promote Health?* New York: Oxford University Press; 2005.

34. Mueller NB, Luke DA, Herbers SH, Montgomery TP. The best practices: use of the guidelines by ten state tobacco control programs. *American Journal of Preventive Medicine* 2006;31(4):300–306.

35. Eriksen, M. Lessons learned from public health efforts and their relevance to preventing childhood obesity. In: Koplan JP, Liverman CT, Kraak VA, editors. *Preventing Childhood Obesity: Health in the Balance*. Washington, DC: National Academy of Sciences; 2005:343-375.

36. National Cancer Institute. *Greater Than the Sum: Systems Thinking in Tobacco Control*. Tobacco Control Monograph No. 18. Bethesda, MD: U.S. Department of Health and Human Services, National Institutes of Health, National Cancer Institute; 2007. NIH Pub No. 06-6085.

37. Federal Trade Commission. *Cigarette Report for 2004 and 2005*. Washington, DC: Federal Trade Commission; 2007.

38. Substance Abuse and Mental Health Services Administration, Office of Applied Studies, National Survey on Drug Use and Health, 2005 and 2006, Table 4.3B. Available at http://oas.samhsa.gov/NSDUH/2k6nsduh/tabs/Sect4peTabs1to4.pdf.

39. California Environmental Protection Agency. *Proposed Identification of Environmental Tobacco Smoke as a Toxic Air Contaminant*. Sacramento: Environmental Protection Agency, Office of Environmental Health Hazard Assessment; 2005.

Section A

I State and Community Interventions

Justification

The history of successful public health practice has demonstrated that the active and coordinated involvement of a wide range of societal and community resources must be the foundation of sustained solutions to pervasive problems like tobacco use.[1-5] In the evidence-based review of population-based tobacco prevention and control efforts, the Task Force on Community Preventive Services confirmed the importance of coordinated and combined intervention efforts.[6] The strongest evidence demonstrating the effectiveness of many of the population-based approaches that are most highly recommended by the Task Force comes from studies in which specific strategies for smoking cessation and prevention of initiation are combined with efforts to mobilize communities and integrate these strategies into synergistic and multi-component efforts.[6] Additionally, research has demonstrated the importance of community support and involvement at the grassroots level in implementing several of the most highly effective policy interventions, such as increasing the unit price of tobacco products and creating smoke-free environments.[3,4,7,8] Example program and policy recommendations from the Task Force, as well as the *Healthy People 2010* policy goals for the nation are provided in Appendix C. The community-based intervention model to create a social and legal climate "in which tobacco becomes less desirable, less acceptable, and less accessible" has now become a core element of statewide comprehensive tobacco control programs.[3,4,7,9-11]

The CDC-recommended comprehensive statewide tobacco control program combines and coordinates community-based interventions that focus on 1) preventing initiation of tobacco use among youth and young adults, 2) promoting quitting among adults and youth, 3) eliminating exposure to secondhand smoke, and 4) identifying and eliminating tobacco-related disparities among population groups. Reducing tobacco use is particularly challenging because tobacco products are so highly addictive. To quote the tobacco industry, "Smoke is beyond question the most optimized vehicle of nicotine and the cigarette the most optimized dispenser of smoke."[12] Additionally, the tobacco industry spends billions of dollars annually to make tobacco use appear to be attractive as well as an accepted and established part of American culture. In addition to these tobacco advertising and promotion campaigns, both adults and youth have been and continue to be heavily exposed to images of smoking in the movies and other mass media.[13-16] Effectively countering these pervasive pro-tobacco influences and helping people stop using these highly addictive tobacco products requires the coordinated implementation of a broad range of statewide and community level programs and policies to influence societal organizations, systems, and networks that encourage and support individuals to make behavior choices consistent with tobacco-free norms.[3,4,9,17,18]

The CDC-recommended community-based model to produce durable changes in social norms is based on evidence that approaches with the greatest span (economic, regulatory, and comprehensive) will have the greatest population impact.[3,4,7,19-21] Recommendations from evidence-based reviews indicate that more individually focused educational and clinical approaches with a smaller span of impact should be combined with population-based efforts at the state and community levels.[3,4,6,7,19]

The budget guidelines in *Best Practices for Comprehensive Tobacco Control Programs— August 1999* included several program elements that are presented here as a single, more integrated component and funding stream.[22] Based on the practice-based model now being implemented in many states, this more integrated program component combines local and statewide policies and programs, chronic disease and tobacco-related disparity elimination initiatives, and interventions specifically aimed at influencing youth.[11]

State and Community Interventions

Statewide Programs

Statewide programs can provide the skills, resources, and information needed for the coordinated, strategic implementation of effective community programs. For example, training local community coalitions about the legal and technical aspects of smoke-free air ordinances and enforcement can be provided most efficiently through statewide partners who have experience in providing these services. Direct funding provided to statewide organizations can be used to mobilize their organizational assets to strengthen community resources.

Each state's financial and social demographic characteristics have a significant role in their tobacco prevention and control efforts. Statewide efforts should include:

• Supporting and/or facilitating tobacco prevention and control coalition development as well as links to other related coalitions (e.g., cancer control)

• Establishing a strategic plan for comprehensive tobacco control with appropriate partners at the state and local levels

• Implementing evidence-based policy interventions to decrease tobacco use initiation, increase cessation, and protect people from exposure to secondhand smoke

• Collecting community-specific data and developing and implementing culturally appropriate interventions with appropriate multicultural involvement

• Sponsoring local, regional, and statewide training, conferences, and technical assistance on best practices for effective tobacco use prevention and cessation programs

• Monitoring pro-tobacco influences to facilitate public discussion and debate among partners, decision makers, and other stakeholders at the community level

• Supporting innovative demonstration and research projects to prevent youth tobacco use, promote cessation, promote tobacco-free communities, and reach diverse populations

Community Programs

A "community" encompasses a diverse set of entities, including voluntary health agencies; civic, social, and recreational organizations; businesses and business associations; city and county governments; public health organizations; labor groups; health care systems and providers; health care professionals' societies; schools and universities; faith communities; and organizations for racial and ethnic minority groups.[1-5,7]

To counter aggressive pro-tobacco influences, communities must become more involved in the way tobacco is promoted, sold, and used while changing the knowledge, attitudes, and practices of tobacco users and nonusers.[4,5] Effective community programs involve and influence people in their homes, work sites, schools, places of worship, places of entertainment, health care settings, civic organizations, and other public places.[1,3-5,23] Changing policies that can influence societal organizations, systems, and networks necessitates the involvement of community partners.[1,2,4] Decreasing disparities in tobacco use occurs largely through community interventions.

State program involvement in community-level interventions should include:

• Providing funding to community-based organizations in order to strengthen the capacity of these groups to positively influence social norms regarding tobacco use and to build relationships between health departments and grassroots, voluntary efforts

• Empowering local agencies to build community coalitions that facilitate collaboration among programs in local governments, voluntary and civic organizations, and diverse community-based organizations

• Collaborating with partners and other programs to implement evidence-based interventions and build and sustain capacity through technical assistance and training

• Supporting local strategies or efforts to educate the public and media not only about the health effects of tobacco use and exposure to secondhand smoke, but also about available cessation services

Community-level Interventions (Continued):
- Promoting public discussion among partners, decision makers, and other stakeholders about tobacco-related health issues and pro-tobacco influences
- Establishing a local strategic plan of action that is consistent with the state's strategic plan
- Ensuring that funding formulas for the local public health infrastructure provide grantees (e.g., local and county health departments, tribal organizations, nonprofit organizations) operating expenses commensurate with tobacco control program and evaluation efforts
- Ensuring that local grantees measure and evaluate social norm change outcomes (e.g., policy adoption, increased compliance) resulting from their interventions

In an effort to identify and eliminate tobacco-related disparities, state programs should:
- Conduct a population assessment to guide efforts
- Seek consultation from specific population groups, tribes, and community-based organizations
- Ensure that disparity issues are an integral part of state and local tobacco control strategic plan
- Provide funding to organizations that can effectively reach, involve, and mobilize identified specific populations
- Provide culturally competent technical assistance and training to grantees and partners
- Provide health communications to address tobacco-related disparities in appropriate languages that support community-level interventions
- Ensure that quitline services are culturally competent and have adequate reach and intensity to meet the required needs of population subgroups

Tobacco-Related Disparities

Because some populations experience a disproportionate health and economic burden from tobacco use, a focus on eliminating such tobacco-related disparities is necessary. Tobacco-related disparities are "differences in patterns, prevention, and treatment of tobacco use; differences in the risk, incidence, morbidity, mortality, and burden of tobacco-related illness that exist among specific population groups in the United States; and related differences in capacity and infrastructure, access to resources, and environmental tobacco smoke exposure."[24] Measuring these characteristics in a population assessment will specifically identify the populations with tobacco-related disparities within a state or community.

State capacity and infrastructure, including clear leadership and dedicated resources, are essential to the development and implementation of a strong strategic plan that includes the identification and elimination of tobacco-related disparities. Reaching the national *Healthy People 2010* goal of eliminating health disparities related to tobacco use will necessitate improved collection and use of standardized and qualitative data to identify disparities in both health outcomes and efficacy of prevention programs among various population groups.[7]

The Washington State Department of Health (WA DOH) provides one example of work in this area. They identified six critical issues to identify and eliminate tobacco-related disparities: "build and sustain [WA] DOH's commitment to identify and eliminate tobacco-related health disparities, build and sustain community and systems capacity to improve access and outreach to underserved communities, make tobacco use a higher priority issue in underserved communities, develop and provide culturally and linguistically appropriate approaches and materials, identify and use culturally sensitive policies and practices, and reduce tobacco industry influence."[25] Since 2003, the program has focused on ways to address these six critical issues and the program's four overarching goals by using a comprehensive approach that includes community and schools, health communication, policy, and evaluation strategies. To date, key outcomes include an ongoing community advisory committee, contracts with organizations in diverse communities and tribes, enhanced data gathering, and the program's first data report on disparities in adult tobacco use; systems change in the state tobacco quitline, Medicaid, Head Start, health care and chemical dependency systems; and increased cultural competency in producing communication and educational materials and in implementing program activities. As a result, WA DOH has used these data to identify specific populations, expand partnerships, and redirect resources to better serve those with the greatest need.[25,26]

The California Smoker's Helpline provides cessation services and culturally appropriate information in multiple languages for different audiences. These focused tobacco cessation interventions have led to significant reductions in smoking across ethnic groups in California. For instance, from 1990 to 2005, smoking rates among Asian men dropped from 20% to less than 15%; among Hispanic men, from 22% to 16%; and among African American men, from 28% to 21%.[27]

The New York tobacco control program has identified populations with chemical addictions or mental illness as having disproportionately high rates of tobacco use. To reach these populations, the state used strategies that included integrating tobacco dependence treatment into treatment protocols for mental illness or chemical dependency, promoting tobacco-free campuses for substance abuse and mental health facilities, and partnering with agencies representing these groups.[28] The Vermont tobacco disparities plan targets smokers who also have mental health and/or substance abuse issues along with smokers with household incomes below 250% of the poverty level. To accomplish this, Vermont is creating and enhancing partnerships with those agencies working with the identified groups and implementing strategies in these agencies to make referrals to existing services. Questions regarding mental health are included in statewide surveys of risk behaviors to continue assessing impact in this population.[29]

CDC has been providing technical assistance and training to state tobacco control programs on how to develop and implement strategic plans to address issues of disparity within the respective states. For more information on how to identify and eliminate tobacco-related disparities, see Appendix D.

Youth

Interventions to prevent tobacco use initiation and encourage cessation among young people need to reshape the environment so that it supports tobacco-free norms. Because most people who start smoking are younger than 18 years of age, intervening during adolescence is critical. Community programs and school-based policies and interventions should be part of a comprehensive effort,

implemented in coordination across the community and school environments and in conjunction with increasing the unit price of tobacco products, sustaining anti-tobacco media campaigns, making environments smoke-free, and engaging in other efforts to create tobacco-free social norms.[6,13,19]

To prevent tobacco use among youth, the independent Task Force on Community Preventive Services' *Guide to Community Preventive Services* recommends:[6,30]

- Increasing the unit price of tobacco products
- Conducting mass media education campaigns when combined with other community interventions
- Mobilizing the community to restrict minors' access to tobacco products when combined with additional interventions (stronger local laws directed at retailers, active enforcement of retailer sales laws, retailer education with reinforcement)
- Implementing school-based interventions in combination with mass media campaigns and additional community efforts

At the time that *Best Practices—2007* went to press, CDC's Division of Adolescent and School Health was updating *School Health Guidelines to Prevent Tobacco Use, Addiction, and Exposure to Secondhand Smoke,* which features policies and strategies most likely to be effective in preventing tobacco use and addiction among young people.[31] *School Health Index: A Self-Assessment and Planning Guide* helps schools assess and improve their health and safety policies and programs in the context of a coordinated school health program.[32] These guidance and assessment tools highlight a comprehensive approach toward eliminating tobacco use initiation by linking schools with the broader community and using policy change as the underpinning to support education and intervention efforts. Another key document—*Fit, Healthy, and Ready to Learn: A School Health Policy Guide*—provides a comprehensive guide to tobacco-free policies and their development.[33]

State and Community Interventions

Chronic Disease Programs

State-based tobacco prevention and control programs can collaborate with other programs to address diseases for which tobacco is a major cause, including multiple cancers, heart disease and stroke, and chronic lung and respiratory diseases. Addressing tobacco control strategies in the broader context of tobacco-related diseases is beneficial for three reasons. First, it is critical that interventions are implemented to alleviate the existing burden of disease from tobacco. Second, the incorporation of tobacco prevention and cessation messages into broader public health activities ensures wider dissemination of tobacco control strategies. Finally, tobacco use in conjunction with other diseases and risk factors, such as sedentary lifestyle, poor diet, and diabetes, poses a greater combined risk for many chronic diseases than the sum of each individual degree of risk. Collaboration in these areas has potential to synergistically increase reach and desired outcomes in states.

Examples of activities to reduce the burden of tobacco-related diseases include the following:

- Collaborating with related public health programs on shared goals and objectives
- Implementing community interventions that link tobacco control interventions, such as smoke-free policies with cardiovascular disease and cancer prevention programs
- Developing counter-marketing strategies to increase awareness of secondhand smoke as a trigger for asthma and an increased risk for heart attacks
- Using tobacco excise tax dollars to fund both tobacco prevention and control and chronic disease prevention and treatment
- Linking chronic disease management programs for diabetes and cardiovascular disease to the state tobacco cessation quitline
- Promoting insurance coverage for a package of preventive services, including high blood pressure, high cholesterol, and tobacco use treatment

CDC's Division for Heart Disease and Stroke Prevention has developed *A Public Health Action Plan to Prevent Heart Disease and Stroke* and supporting guidance materials to provide public health professionals and decision makers with targeted recommendations and specific action steps to reverse the trend in heart disease and stroke through effective prevention.[34] Guidance materials include *Translating the Public Health Action Plan into Action* and *Moving into Action: Promoting Heart-Healthy and Stroke-Free Communities*.[35,36]

CDC's Division of Cancer Prevention and Control's National Comprehensive Cancer Control Program funds 50 states, the District of Columbia, seven territories, and seven tribes or tribal-serving organizations to develop and implement comprehensive cancer control plans. The Division has developed *Guidance for Comprehensive Cancer Control Planning,* which includes a guideline and a toolkit for implementing and evaluating a comprehensive cancer control plan.[37] In addition, the Cancer Control P.L.A.N.E.T. website provides links to comprehensive cancer control resources, including tobacco control activities.[38]

CDC's Division of Diabetes Translation has made smoking prevention and cessation for people with diabetes a major program goal. At the time *Best Practices—2007* went to press, the Division of Diabetes Translation, in collaboration with CDC's Office on Smoking and Health, was in the process of identifying best practices pertinent to people with diabetes as well as measures to monitor and evaluate smoking prevalence and cessation among people with diabetes.

Colorado provides an example of implementing a more integrated chronic disease prevention and tobacco control program. The objectives from the state's tobacco prevention and control strategic plan have been incorporated into Colorado's Cancer Plan and Cardiovascular Plan. Cancer, cardiovascular disease, asthma, and diabetes interventions reflect the relationship between smoking and each disease by including promotion of the state's quitline; asthma messages also were integrated into a recent Secondhand Smoke and Children campaign that encouraged calls to the state's quitline. In 2004, a Colorado voter referendum secured all new tobacco excise tax revenues for health initiatives, including chronic disease programs that address cancer, heart disease, and lung diseases; tobacco prevention and control; and expansion of Medicaid and the Children's Health Insurance Program, community health centers, and the Old Age Pension Fund.[39]

Budget

Linking state and community interventions creates synergistic effects, greatly increasing the effects of each of the program's individual components. Policy discussions, youth programs, health communication interventions, and cessation interventions all serve to reinforce one another. Evidence indicates that implementing policies that promote a change in social norms appear to be the most effective approach for sustained behavior change.[6]

Best practices dictate allocating funds for establishing and sustaining internal capacity with experienced staff and developing an infrastructure with partner organizations and other programs to oversee and implement evidence-based programs. Most states fund local health departments, boards of health, or health-related nonprofit community organizations representing each county or major metropolitan area to develop and maintain local infrastructure and implement population-based and targeted programs. Funds are also awarded directly to tribal health departments and tribal-serving organizations and other community-based organizations that serve specific populations for implementing evidence-based programs and activities. Funds may also be distributed to different agencies on the basis of who is responsible for enforcing tobacco prevention and control laws. These varied efforts remain integrated through good communication, coalitions, and networks. States should take into account the special issues of different communities within their state, such as large variations in population size, differences in prevalence in various populations, and reach of the interventions.

Recommendations for funding State and Community Interventions are based on the 1999 funding formulas for Statewide Programs, Community Programs to Reduce Tobacco Use, Chronic Disease Programs to Reduce the Burden of Tobacco-Related Diseases, School Programs, and Enforcement.[22] The recommended range of funding is derived from the sum of the 1999 funding formulas, adjusted for population changes and inflation. The specific state-recommended level of investment within that range is based on the relative complexity and cost of doing business in that state. Drawing from the experience of states that have implemented robust state and community interventions, a recommended funding level was applied to states. For the Statewide Programs and Community Programs funding ranges, the recommended level of investment was based primarily on each state's current smoking prevalence, while also taking into account other factors, such as the proportion of individuals within the state living at or below 200% of the poverty level; average wage rates for implementing public health programs; the state's infrastructure (as reflected by the number of governmental health units with a jurisdiction smaller than the state); and geographic size. Because the science base supporting how to best implement chronic disease programs integrated with tobacco control and some youth interventions (e.g., empowerment programs) is still evolving, their portion of the recommended level of investment was based on the 1999 minimum base and per capita recommendations, adjusted for inflation.

Since 1999, states have adapted the CDC recommendations based on state dynamics and to meet particular needs. Priority activities should focus on those with the greatest impact and proven level of efficacy as well as those that build on the success of other evidence-based interventions. [6,7,19]

I State and Community Interventions

Core Resources

California Department of Health Services. *A Model for Change: The California Experience in Tobacco Control.* Sacramento: California Department of Health Services; 1998. Available at http://www.dhs.ca.gov/tobacco/documents/pubs/modelforchange.pdf.

California Department of Health Services. *Communities of Excellence in Tobacco Control.* Sacramento: California Department of Health Services, Tobacco Control Section; 2006. Available at http://www.dhs.ca.gov/tobacco/html/publications htm#cx2006.

Tobacco Technical Assistance Consortium. *Communities of Excellence Plus.* Available at http://www.ttac.org/trainings/pdfs/CX_Plus.pdf.

National Cancer Institute. *ASSIST: Shaping the Future of Tobacco Prevention and Control.* Tobacco Control Monograph No. 16. Bethesda, MD: U.S. Department of Health and Human Services, National Institutes of Health, National Cancer Institute; 2005. NIH Pub. No. 05-5645. Available at http://cancercontrol.cancer.gov/tcrb/monographs/16/index html.

National Cancer Institute. *Evaluating ASSIST: A Blueprint for Understanding State-Level Tobacco Control.* Tobacco Control Monograph No. 17. Bethesda, MD: U.S. Department of Health and Human Services, National Institutes of Health, National Cancer Institute; 2006. NIH Pub. No.06-6058. Available at http://cancercontrol.cancer.gov/tcrb/monographs/17/index.html.

U.S. Department of Health and Human Services. *Reducing Tobacco Use: A Report of the Surgeon General.* Atlanta: U.S. Department of Health and Human Services, Centers for Disease Control and Prevention, National Center for Chronic Disease Prevention and Health Promotion, Office on Smoking and Health; 2000. Available at http://www.cdc.gov/tobacco/data_statistics/sgr/sgr_2000/index.htm.

U.S. Department of Health and Human Services. *The Health Consequences of Involuntary Exposure to Tobacco Smoke: A Report of the Surgeon General.* Atlanta: U.S. Department of Health and Human Services, Centers for Disease Control and Prevention, Coordinating Center for Health Promotion, National Center for Chronic Disease Prevention and Health Promotion, Office on Smoking and Health; 2006. Available at http://www.cdc.gov/tobacco/data_statistics/sgr/sgr_2006/index.htm.

Zaza S, Briss PA, Harris KW, editors. *The Guide to Community Preventive Services: What Works to Promote Health?* New York: Oxford University Press; 2005. Available at http://www.thecommunityguide.org/tobacco/default.htm.

Institute of Medicine. *Ending the Tobacco Problem: A Blueprint for the Nation.* Washington, DC: National Academies Press; 2007.

National Cancer Institute. Tobacco use prevention and treatment. In: *Promoting Healthy Lifestyles: Policy, Program, and Personal Recommendations for Reducing Cancer Risk—2006–2007 Annual Report, President's Cancer Panel.* Bethesda, MD: U.S. Department of Health and Human Services, National Institutes of Health, National Cancer Institute; 2007:61-92. Available at http://deainfo.nci nih.gov/advisory/pcp/pcp07rpt/pcp07rpt.pdf.

Starr G, Rogers T, Schooley M, Porter S, Wiesen E, Jamison N. *Key Outcome Indicators for Evaluating Comprehensive Tobacco Control Programs.* Atlanta: Centers for Disease Control and Prevention; 2005. Available at http://www.cdc.gov/tobacco/tobacco_control_programs/surveillance_evaluation/key_outcome/index htm.

U.S. Department of Health and Human Services. *Tobacco Use Among U.S. Racial/Ethnic Minority Groups—African Americans, American Indians and Alaska Natives, Asian Americans and Pacific Islanders, and Hispanics: A Report of the Surgeon General.* Atlanta: U.S. Department of Health and Human Services, Centers for Disease Control and Prevention, National Center for Chronic Disease Prevention and Health Promotion, Office on Smoking and Health; 1998. Available at http://www.cdc.gov/tobacco/data_statistics/sgr/sgr_1998/index htm.

U.S. Department of Health and Human Services. *Preventing Tobacco Use Among Young People: A Report of the Surgeon General.* Atlanta: U.S. Department of Health and Human Services, Public Health Service, Centers for Disease Control and Prevention, National Center for Chronic Disease Prevention and Health Promotion, Office on Smoking and Health; 1994. Available at http://www.cdc.gov/tobacco/data_statistics/sgr/sgr_1994/index htm.

Centers for Disease Control and Prevention. *School Health Guidelines to Prevent Tobacco Use, Addiction, and Exposure to Secondhand Smoke.* Atlanta: Centers for Disease Control and Prevention. In progress.

Centers for Disease Control and Prevention. *School Health Index: A Self-Assessment and Planning Guide.* Elementary or middle school/high school version. Atlanta: Centers for Disease Control and Prevention; 2005. Available at http://apps nccd.cdc.gov/shi/default.aspx.

National Association of State Boards of Education. *Fit, Healthy, and Ready to Learn: A School Health Policy Guide.* Atlanta: Centers for Disease Control and Prevention; 2007. Available at http://www.nasbe.org/healthy_schools/FHRTL.htm.

Substance Abuse and Mental Health Services Administration. Final regulations to implement section 1926 of the Public Health Service Act regarding the sale and distribution of tobacco products to individuals under the age of 18. *Federal Register* 1996;13:1492–1500. Available at http://frwebgate.access.gpo.gov/cgi-bin/getpage.cgi?dbname=1996_register&position=all&page=1492.

Substance Abuse and Mental Health Services Administration. *Synar Regulation: Tobacco Outlet Inspection-Guidance.* Rockville, MD: SAMHSA, Center for Substance Abuse Prevention; 1997.

Partnership for Prevention, National Association of Chronic Disease Directors. *Comprehensive and Integrated Chronic Disease Prevention: Action Planning Handbook for States and Communities.* Washington, DC: Partnership for Prevention; 2005. Available at http://www.prevent.org/images/stories/action_planning_handbook.pdf.

Partnership for Prevention. *Chronic Disease Prevention: Action Planning for States and Communities: Case Studies.* Washington, DC: Partnership for Prevention; 2005. Available at http://www.prevent.org/images/stories/Files/publications/casestudies.pdf.

Centers for Disease Control and Prevention. *A Public Health Action Plan to Prevent Heart Disease and Stroke.* Atlanta: U.S. Department of Health and Human Services, Centers for Disease Control and Prevention; 2003. Available at http://www.cdc.gov/dhdsp/library/action_plan/index.htm#executive.

Centers for Disease Control and Prevention. *A Public Health Action Plan to Prevent Heart Disease and Stroke: Translating the Plan into Action.* Atlanta: U.S. Department of Health and Human Services, Centers for Disease Control and Prevention; 2004. Available at http://www.cdc.gov/dhdsp/library/action_plan/Update/.

Centers for Disease Control and Prevention. *Moving into Action: Promoting Heart–Healthy and Stroke–Free Communities.* Atlanta: U.S. Department of Health and Human Services; 2005. Available at http://www.cdc.gov/dhdsp/library/moving_into_action/order.htm.

Centers for Disease Control and Prevention. *Guidance for Comprehensive Cancer Control Planning. Volume I: Guidelines. Volume 2: Toolkit.* Atlanta: Centers for Disease Control and Prevention; 2002. Available at http://www.cdc.gov/cancer/ncccp/.

Centers for Disease Control and Prevention. Cancer Control Plan, Link, Act, Network with Evidence-based Tools (P.L.A.N.E.T.). Available at http://cancercontrolplanet.cancer.gov.

Centers for Disease Control and Prevention. Smoking & Tobacco Use website. Available at www.cdc.gov/tobacco.

I State and Community Interventions

References

1. Green LW, Kreuter M. *Health Promotion Planning: An Educational and Ecological Approach.* New York: McGraw-Hill; 2000.

2. Institute of Medicine. *The Future of Public's Health in the 21ˢᵗ Century.* Washington, DC: National Academies Press; 2002.

3. Eriksen, M. Lessons learned from public health efforts and their relevance to preventing childhood obesity. In: Koplan JP, Liverman CT, Kraak VA, editors. *Preventing Childhood Obesity: Health in the Balance.* Washington, DC: National Academy of Sciences; 2005:343-375.

4. National Cancer Institute. *ASSIST: Shaping the Future of Tobacco Prevention and Control.* Tobacco Control Monograph No. 16. Bethesda, MD: U.S. Department of Health and Human Services, National Institutes of Health, National Cancer Institute; 2005. NIH Pub No. 05-5645.

5. Cummings KM, Sciandra R, Carol J, Burgess S, Tye JB, Flewelling R. Approaches directed to the social environment. In: *Strategies to Control Tobacco Use in the United States: A Blueprint for Public Health in the 1990's.* Tobacco Control Monograph No. 1. Washington, DC: U.S. Department of Health and Human Services; 1991:203–265.

6. Zaza S, Briss PA, Harris KW, editors. *The Guide to Community Preventive Services: What Works to Promote Health?* New York: Oxford University Press; 2005.

7. U.S. Department of Health and Human Services. *Reducing Tobacco Use: A Report of the Surgeon General.* Atlanta: U.S. Department of Health and Human Services, Centers for Disease Control and Prevention, National Center for Chronic Disease Prevention and Health Promotion, Office on Smoking and Health; 2000.

8. U.S. Department of Health and Human Services. *The Health Consequences of Involuntary Exposure to Tobacco Smoke: A Report of the Surgeon General.* Atlanta: U.S. Department of Health and Human Services, Centers for Disease Control and Prevention, Coordinating Center for Health Promotion, National Center for Chronic Disease Prevention and Health Promotion, Office on Smoking and Health; 2006.

9. California Department of Health Services. *A Model for Change: The California Experience in Tobacco Control.* Sacramento: California Department of Health Services; 1998.

10. National Cancer Institute. *Evaluating ASSIST: A Blueprint for Understanding State-Level Tobacco Control.* Tobacco Control Monograph No. 17. Bethesda, MD: U.S. Department of Health and Human Services, National Institutes of Health, National Cancer Institute; 2006. NIH Pub No. 06-6058.

11. Mueller NB, Luke DA, Herbers SH, Montgomery TP. The best practices: use of the guidelines by ten state tobacco control programs. *American Journal of Preventive Medicine* 2006;31:300–306.

12. Dunn WL. *Motives and Incentives in Cigarette Smoking.* Richmond, VA: Philip Morris Research Center; 1972.

13. U.S. Department of Health and Human Services. *Preventing Tobacco Use Among Young People: A Report of the Surgeon General.* Atlanta: U.S. Department of Health and Human Services, Public Health Service, Centers for Disease Control and Prevention, National Center for Chronic Disease Prevention and Health Promotion, Office on Smoking and Health; 1994.

14. Charlesworth A, Glantz SA. Tobacco and the movie industry. *Clinics in Occupational and Environmental Medicine* 2006;5(1):73–84.

15. Cummings KM, Morley CP, Horan JK, Leavell N-R. Marketing to America's youth: evidence from corporate documents. *Tobacco Control* 2002;11 (Suppl 1):i5-i17.

16. Sargent JD, Stoolmiller M, Worth KA, Dal Cin S, Wills TA, Gibbons FX, et al. Exposure to smoking depictions in movies: Its association with established adolescent smoking. *Archives of Pediatric Adolescent Medicine* 2007;161(9):849-856.

17. California Department of Health Services. *Communities of Excellence in Tobacco Control.* Sacramento: California Department of Health Services, Tobacco Control Section; 2006.

18. Tobacco Technical Assistance Consortium. *Communities of Excellence Plus.* Available at http://www.ttac.org/trainings/pdfs/CX_Plus.pdf.

19. Institute of Medicine. *Ending the Tobacco Problem: A Blueprint for the Nation.* Washington, DC: National Academies Press; 2007.

20. Brownson RC, Haire-Joshu D, Luke DA. Shaping the context of health: a review of environmental and policy approaches in the prevention of chronic disease. *Annual Review of Public Health* 2006;27:341-370.

21. Wisotzky M, Albuquerque M, Pechacek TF, Park BZ. The National Tobacco Control Program: Focusing on policy to broaden impact. *Public Health Reports* 2004;119:303-310.

22. Centers for Disease Control and Prevention. *Best Practices for Comprehensive Tobacco Control Programs—August 1999.* Atlanta: U.S. Department of Health and Human Services; 1999.

23. Minkler M, editor. *Community Organizing and Community Building for Health.* 2nd edition. New Brunswick, NJ: Rutgers University Press; 2005.

24. Fagan P, King G, Lawrence D, Petrucci SA, Robinson RG, Banks D, et al. Eliminating tobacco-related health disparities: directions for future research. *American Journal of Public Health* 2004;94:211–217.

25. Washington State Department of Health. *Adult Smoking Rates in Washington: A Report on Current Disparities.* Olympia, WA: Washington State Department of Health; 2007.

26. Washington State Department of Health. *Strategic Plan for Identifying and Eliminating Tobacco-Related Health Disparities in Washington State.* Olympia, WA: Washington State Department of Health; 2004.

27. California Department of Health Services. California releases new data and anti-smoking ads targeting diverse populations. News Release No. 06-82, October 2, 2006. Available at http://www.dhs.ca.gov/ tobacco/documents/press/PR-October-2006.pdf.

28. New York State Department of Health. Cooperative Agreement Interim Progress Report. Unpublished report submitted to CDC, February 9, 2007.

29. Vermont Department of Health. Cooperative Agreement Interim Progress Report. Unpublished report submitted to CDC, January 17, 2007.

30. Task Force on Community Preventive Services. Recommendations regarding interventions to reduce tobacco use and exposure to environmental tobacco smoke. *American Journal of Preventive Medicine* 2001;20(2S):10–15.

31. Centers for Disease Control and Prevention. *School Health Guidelines to Prevent Tobacco Use, Addiction, and Exposure to Secondhand Smoke.* Atlanta: Centers for Disease Control and Prevention. In progress.

32. Centers for Disease Control and Prevention. *School Health Index: A Self-Assessment and Planning Guide.* Elementary or middle school/high school version. Atlanta: Centers for Disease Control and Prevention; 2005.

33. National Association of State Boards of Education. *Fit, Healthy, and Ready to Learn: A School Health Policy Guide.* Atlanta: Centers for Disease Control and Prevention; 2007.

34. Centers for Disease Control and Prevention. *A Public Health Action Plan to Prevent Heart Disease and Stroke.* Atlanta: U.S. Department of Health and Human Services; 2003.

35. Centers for Disease Control and Prevention. *A Public Health Action Plan to Prevent Heart Disease and Stroke: Translating the Plan into Action.* Atlanta: U.S. Department of Health and Human Services; 2004.

36. Centers for Disease Control and Prevention. *Moving into Action: Promoting Heart–Healthy and Stroke–Free Communities.* Atlanta: U.S. Department of Health and Human Services; 2005.

37. Centers for Disease Control and Prevention. *Guidance for Comprehensive Cancer Control Planning. Volume I: Guidelines. Volume 2: Toolkit.* Atlanta: Centers for Disease Control and Prevention; 2002.

38. Centers for Disease Control and Prevention. Cancer Control Plan, Link, Act, Network with Evidence-based Tools (P.L.A.N.E.T.). Available at http:// cancercontrolplanet.cancer.gov.

39. Colorado Department of Public Health and Environment. *Making a Difference in Colorado's Health: A Report on the Colorado Department of Public Health and Environment Programs Funded by Amendment 35.* Denver, CO: Colorado Department of Public Health and Environment; 2007.

Health Communication Interventions

Justification

Health communication interventions can be powerful tools for preventing smoking initiation, promoting and facilitating cessation, and shaping social norms related to tobacco use. Effective messages that are targeted appropriately can stimulate public support for tobacco control interventions and create a supportive climate for policy and programmatic community efforts.[1] The independent Task Force on Community Preventive Services' *Guide to Community Preventive Services* strongly recommends sustained media campaigns, combined with other interventions and strategies, as an effective strategy to decrease the likelihood of tobacco initiation and promote smoking cessation.[2]

Background

Billions of dollars are spent annually by tobacco companies to make tobacco use appear to be attractive as well as an accepted and established part of American culture. These tobacco advertising and promotion activities do much more—substantial evidence indicates that the tobacco manufacturers compete vigorously with each other for a share of the youth market.[3-5] For more than two decades, the three most heavily advertised brands (Marlboro, Newport, and Camel) have accounted for more than 80% of brands smoked by adolescents.[6-9]

Social norms play a significant role in shaping beliefs and behaviors in healthy and unhealthy ways.[10] For example, survey data from California indicate that adult smokers with strong attitudes about the health effects and restriction of secondhand smoke are more than twice as likely to have made a recent quit attempt and to have the intention to quit in the next six months.[11] Adult smokers who demonstrated strong anti-tobacco industry beliefs were 65% more likely to have made a recent quit attempt and 85% more likely to have the intention to quit in the next six months.[11]

Adolescents and young adults are very sensitive to perceived social norms and media presentations of smoking behavior.[12,13] Nonsmoking adolescents exposed to tobacco advertising and promotional campaigns are significantly more likely to become young adult smokers.[14,15] Because adolescents and young adults have been and continue to be so heavily exposed to images of smoking in the media, tobacco advertising, and promotional campaigns, public health counter-marketing campaigns are needed to focus on preventing initiation and promoting cessation.

In 1998, the tobacco industry settled a lawsuit with 46 states to recoup funding from Medicaid expenses resulting from the treatment of tobacco-related illness, after having settled with four states individually.[1] This multi-state Master Settlement Agreement (MSA) included specific tobacco industry restrictions related to youth access, marketing, lobbying, and some types of outdoor advertising. After the settlement, tobacco marketing expenditures more than doubled over the next five years. In 2005, tobacco companies spent $13.4 billion to market cigarettes and smokeless tobacco, outspending the nation's total tobacco prevention and cessation efforts by a ratio of more than 22 to 1.[16,17] Although the majority of current tobacco marketing consists of price discounts (which offset the anticipated impact of excise tax increases on tobacco consumption and on youth and adult prevalence), tobacco company traditional advertising budgets still exceed spending on public health-sponsored anti-tobacco campaigns.[16-20] Since the MSA, tobacco promotions have shifted away from traditional media (e.g., billboards and magazines) and moved toward retail outlets.[21] Research indicates that point-of-sale advertising is associated with encouraging youth, particularly younger teens, to try smoking and that cigarette promotions are more influential with youth already experimenting with cigarettes as they progress to regular smoking.[20] Furthermore, youth- and parent-focused anti-tobacco advertising campaigns sponsored by the tobacco industry have been shown to actually increase youth tobacco use.[22,23] Youth exposed to these ads are more likely to report greater intention to smoke in the future and more positive feelings toward the tobacco industry than those who were not exposed.[22,23]

Efficacy of Tobacco Counter-Marketing

The Fairness Doctrine campaign of 1967–1970—the first sustained nationwide tobacco control media effort—documented that an intensive mass media campaign can produce significant declines in smoking rates among both adults and youth.[24] A 1999–2000 survey of youth from across the continental United States found that mean exposure to at least one state-sponsored anti-tobacco advertisement in the past four months was associated with greater anti-smoking attitudes and beliefs, such as the perception that smoking is harmful to health and the intention to not smoke in the future.[25] In 2000, the American Legacy Foundation launched truth®, a national campaign to discourage tobacco use among youth, with funding from the MSA. An evaluation of this campaign, which demonstrated the health effects of smoking with graphic images and revealed tobacco industry marketing practices, found it was associated with significant declines in youth smoking prevalence.[26] This evaluation also demonstrated a dose-response relationship between exposure to the truth® campaign and youth smoking, with higher levels of exposure being related to lower prevalence of youth smoking.[26]

Statewide programs—such as those in California, Massachusetts, and Florida—that have featured a variety of interventions, including paid media campaigns, have had the most success in slowing initiation among youth, reducing tobacco use among adults, and protecting the public from the harmful effects of secondhand smoke exposure.[1,27] In the three years after Massachusetts' implementation of a cigarette price increase and robust counter-marketing campaign, adult smoking prevalence decreased 9% (from 23.5% to 21.3%).[28] In just one year, a comprehensive prevention program financed by state settlement dollars and anchored by an aggressive mass media campaign produced significant declines in tobacco use among Florida middle and high school students.[29]

As part of its comprehensive tobacco prevention and control campaign, California has targeted media and local efforts to reach Asian, Hispanic, African American, and American Indian and Alaska Native populations. For example, the state provides targeted promotions of the California Smokers' Helpline, which offers cessation services and information in a variety of languages including English, Spanish, Mandarin, Cantonese, Vietnamese, and Korean. The state has demonstrated success in recruiting target populations to the quitline; in fact, some ethnic minorities are particularly well represented.[30] California's anti-tobacco program has also led to significant reductions in smoking across ethnic groups. For instance, from 1990 to 2005, smoking rates among Asian men dropped from 20% to less than 15%; among Hispanic men, from 22% to 16%; and among African American men, from 28% to 21%.[31]

From 2000 to 2003, Minnesota ran a successful anti-tobacco youth prevention program that featured a continual, high-profile media campaign. However, within six months of the program being dismantled, awareness of the message had eroded and the likelihood of youth to initiate smoking increased from 43% to 53%, providing evidence that sustained media efforts are important.[32]

Beginning in 2002, New York City implemented a multi-pronged, phased initiative to reduce adult and youth smoking rates that included increasing the state's tobacco excise tax, making workplaces smoke-free, expanding cessation services, providing tobacco education, and implementing an extensive television-based media campaign. Ads were broadcast at varying levels for 10 months, with a total exposure over the full campaign of approximately 6,500 gross rating points (GRPs)* (see note at end of section). The state conducted a simultaneous anti-tobacco campaign that resulted in an additional 4,400 GRPs over 12 months for New York City. From 2002 to 2006, adult smoking rates in the city declined 19% overall. Among young adults aged 18 to 24 years, smoking declined 17% in the year after the implementation of the media campaign and 35% from the start of the initiative in 2002.[33]

II Health Communication Interventions

Recommendations

An effective state health communication intervention should deliver strategic, culturally appropriate, and high-impact messages in sustained and adequately funded campaigns integrated into the overall state tobacco program effort.[27] Traditional health communication interventions and counter-marketing strategies employ a wide range of efforts, including paid television, radio, billboard, print, and web-based advertising at the state and local levels; media advocacy through public relations efforts, such as press releases, local events, media literacy, and health promotion activities; and efforts to reduce or replace tobacco industry sponsorship and promotions. Innovations in health communication interventions include targeting specific audiences through personal communication devices (e.g., text messaging) and online networking environments, as well as fostering message development and dissemination by target audience through innovative channels (such as web logs or "blogs").

Behavior theory, audience research, market research, and counter-marketing surveillance are grounded in communication science and are used to develop interventions that target specific audiences (e.g., adults, youth, and disparate populations) with tailored messages that can result in knowledge, attitude, and behavior change. These methods are often used to identify key strategies, influential messages, and the most effective communication channels and media options to reach specific audiences, including diverse and higher-risk populations.

Although the relative effectiveness of specific message concepts and strategies varies by target audience, research from all available sources shows that counter-marketing and other media must have sufficient reach, frequency, and duration to be successful.[34-36] The goal is to reach a defined target audience with fresh and attention-getting messages as efficiently and economically as possible. Media buys are an integral part of an overall strategy. Effective media planning works within the total framework of the campaign's goals. It is estimated that ads should reach 75% to 85% of the target audience each quarter of the year during a media campaign, with an average of 1,200 targeted rating points (TRPs)* (see note at end of section) per quarter during the introduction of a campaign and 800 TRPs per quarter thereafter.[35] While some very well-financed campaigns have exceeded these benchmarks, a campaign should be expected to run at least six months to affect awareness of the issue, 12 to 18 months to have an impact on attitudes, and 18 to 24 months to influence behavior.[35] Campaigns need to overcome pro-tobacco marketing influences, and so reasonable expectations of effectiveness should be set.

The experience of tobacco control campaigns in many states, including Arizona, California, Florida, Massachusetts, Minnesota, and Oregon, as well as the national American Legacy Foundation campaign, suggests that message content is very important. Messages that elicit strong emotional response, such as personal testimonials and viscerally negative content, produce stronger and more consistent effects on audience recall.[36] Aggressive state and national counter-marketing campaigns that have more directly confronted the tobacco industry's marketing tactics have also demonstrated effectiveness but have often become targets for budget cuts.[37]

In addition to providing sufficient reach, frequency, and duration, effective media and health communication intervention efforts should include:

- Audience research to define the thematic characteristics and execution of messages and to develop campaigns that are influential, have high impact, and engage specific audiences
- Market research to not only identify the knowledge, attitudes, and behaviors of target audiences but also the behavioral theory that best motivates specific audiences to change
- Counter-marketing surveillance to understand pro-tobacco messaging, media analysis, and marketing tactics
- Grassroots promotions, local media advocacy, event sponsorships, and other community tie-ins to support and reinforce the statewide campaign and to counter pro-tobacco influences
- Technologies such as viral marketing, social networks, personal web pages, and blogs to generate messages that are then disseminated by the target audience
- Process and outcome evaluation of a comprehensive communication effort as well as specific evaluations of new and innovative approaches
- Promotion of available services, including the state's telephone cessation quitline number or the national portal number (1-800-QUIT NOW)

Planning tools, such as CDC's tobacco control version of *CDCynergy* and *Designing and Implementing an Effective Tobacco Counter-Marketing Campaign,* can be used to systematically plan communication within the larger context of a comprehensive tobacco control program.[27,38] In addition, *Tobacco Counter-Marketing Paid Media Evaluation Manual* (in press) provides evaluators of paid media campaigns with tools to help refine counter-marketing activities and supply results to stakeholders for program accountability and maintenance. *Tobacco Use Prevention Media Campaigns: Lessons Learned from Youth in Nine Countries* provides guidance on the elements of paid media campaigns that have demonstrated effectiveness among young people.[35]

---

* Reach and frequency are the fundamental building blocks for planning and measuring the success of advertising campaigns. *Reach* refers to the number of unduplicated homes/people exposed at least once to a particular ad. *Frequency* is the average number of times a home or individual is exposed to an ad during a given period of time. A rating represents the percent of a specific population group that is exposed to a television or radio program. Each rating point represents 1% of the population the campaign is trying to reach. *Gross rating points* (GRPs) are a measure of the total intensity of a media plan. *Targeted rating points* (TRPs) are used when a specific subpopulation such as 12–17 year olds or 18–44 year olds are targeted.

Reach x Frequency = GRPs. For example, if a campaign reaches 50% of the audience three times (50 x 3) or 75% of the audience two times (75 x 2), either would equal 150 GRPs.

II Health Communication Interventions

Budget

Health communication efforts need to be adequately funded, sustained over time, and integrated with other program activities in order to counter tobacco industry marketing and effectively reduce tobacco use initiation and increase cessation. Campaigns of longer duration and higher intensity are associated with greater declines in smoking rates.[26,39-41] Currently, no sustained federal funding is available for national campaigns. The American Legacy Foundation's truth® and other national campaigns are made possible by the MSA, but future funding for these campaigns remains uncertain. Thus, in the current situation, states need to provide the primary budget for health communication interventions addressing youth prevention, adult cessation, and protection from secondhand smoke to ensure that all state residents will be exposed to messages that address the multiple goals of the comprehensive tobacco control program.

Budget recommendations should be sufficient to conduct a health communication campaign in the state's major media markets addressing cessation (including promotion of the state's quitline), general education about the health hazards of tobacco use and secondhand smoke exposure and youth prevention. Funds should be competitively awarded to firms that understand a state's media markets, have experience in reaching culturally diverse audiences, and have the ability to do market research and counter-marketing surveillance. Additional guidance on selecting contractors for health communication interventions is available in *Designing and Implementing an Effective Tobacco Counter-Marketing Campaign.*[27]

Recommendations for funding Health Communication Interventions are based on the 1999 funding formula for Counter-Marketing. This range of funding was adjusted for changes in inflation and applied to states according to the cost and complexity of their media markets, in part measured by the quantity and coverage provided by a state's designated market areas (DMAs). AC Nielsen cost estimates for buying televised air time in 2006 by state were provided to CDC on November 20, 2006. The specific state-recommended level of investment within the funding range was determined on the basis of the state's relative cost for purchasing 1,200 TRPs per quarter to reach youth aged 12 to 17 years. Comparable relative costs are expected for campaigns that reach other target audiences. This relative cost was then adjusted up or down to reflect the state's effectiveness in reaching 80% of the target population through their recommended DMAs. For example, in Hawaii, all of the target audience lives within one media market and can be reached by purchasing television air time in the local DMA. However, many states have counties that fall outside their primary DMAs, and they may need to consider purchasing media in a neighboring state to reach the minimum recommended level of the target audience. Also, budgeting for effective media campaigns is more complicated for states having media markets that share major metropolitan areas with neighboring states.

Programs of greater intensity using a range of media formats may be needed to tailor the campaign to specific population groups. The cost of audience research, message development, and ad placement will vary significantly across states and media markets. Additional funds may also be required to develop new advertising materials. However, states can lower program development costs by using existing television, radio, print, and outdoor ads from CDC's Media Campaign Resource Center (MCRC), a clearinghouse of high-quality materials produced by states and other organizations.[42] Alternative forms of advertising—such as direct mail; Internet or text-messaging; working through healthcare providers, other government organizations, or media advocacy—can extend the reach of a message, as can recruiting audiences to produce, place, and promote messages themselves through social networks and other web-based technologies.

Core Resources

Zaza S, Briss PA, Harris KW, editors. *The Guide to Community Preventive Services: What Works to Promote Health?* New York: Oxford University Press; 2005. Available at http://www.thecommunityguide.org/tobacco/default.htm.

Centers for Disease Control and Prevention. *Designing and Implementing an Effective Tobacco Counter-Marketing Campaign.* Atlanta: U.S. Department of Health and Human Services; 2003. Available at http://www.cdc.gov/tobacco/media_communications/countermarketing/campaign/index.htm.

Schar E, Gutierrez K, Murphy-Hoefer R, Nelson DE. *Tobacco Use Prevention Media Campaigns: Lessons Learned from Youth in Nine Countries.* Atlanta: U.S. Department of Health and Human Services, Centers for Disease Control and Prevention, National Center for Chronic Disease Prevention and Health Promotion, Office on Smoking and Health; 2006. Available at http://www.cdc.gov/tobacco/youth/00_pdfs/YouthMedia.pdf.

National Cancer Institute. *Making Health Communication Programs Work.* Washington, DC: National Institutes of Health; 2002. Available at http://www.cancer.gov/pinkbook/page1.

National Cancer Institute. *Theory at a Glance: A Guide for Health Promotion Practice.* Washington, DC: National Institutes of Health; 2005. Available at http://www.nci.nih.gov/PDF/481f5d53-63df-41bc-bfaf-5aa48ee1da4d/TAAG3.pdf.

Murphy-Hoefer R, Porter S, Nierderdeppe J, Farrelly M, Sly D, Yarsevich J. *Introduction to Countermarketing Evaluation for Comprehensive Tobacco Control Programs.* Atlanta: Centers for Disease Control and Prevention. In press.

Centers for Disease Control and Prevention. *Telephone Quitlines: A Resource for Development, Implementation, and Evaluation.* Atlanta: U.S. Department of Health and Human Services, Centers for Disease Control and Prevention, National Center for Chronic Disease Prevention and Health Promotion, Office on Smoking and Health; 2004. Available at http://www.cdc.gov/tobacco/quit_smoking/cessation/quitlines/index.htm.

Wallack L, Dorfman L, Jernigan D, Themba M. *Media Advocacy and Public Health.* Newbury Park, CA: Sage Publications; 1993.

Centers for Disease Control and Prevention. Media Campaign Resource Center (MCRC) Online Database. Available at http://www.cdc.gov/tobacco/media_communications/countermarketing/mcrc/index.htm.

Centers for Disease Control and Prevention. CDCynergy, Tobacco Prevention and Control Edition. Available at http://apps.nccd.cdc.gov/osh_pub_catalog/PublicationList.aspx (enter search term "CDCynergy").

Centers for Disease Control and Prevention. Smoking & Tobacco Use website. Available at www.cdc.gov/tobacco.

References

1. U.S. Department of Health and Human Services. *Reducing Tobacco Use: A Report of the Surgeon General.* Atlanta: U.S. Department of Health and Human Services, Centers for Disease Control and Prevention, National Center for Chronic Disease Prevention and Health Promotion, Office on Smoking and Health; 2000.

2. Zaza S, Briss PA, Harris KW, editors. *The Guide to Community Preventive Services: What Works to Promote Health?* New York: Oxford University Press; 2005.

3. U.S. Department of Health and Human Services, Food and Drug Administration. Analysis regarding the Food and Drug Administration's jurisdiction over nicotine-containing cigarettes and smokeless tobacco products. 60 *Federal Register* 1995:41453.

4. U.S. Department of Health and Human Services, Food and Drug Administration. Regulations restricting the sale and distribution of cigarettes and smokeless tobacco to protect children and adolescents. 60 *Federal Register* 1995:41314.

5. Cummings KM, Morley CP, Horan JK, Steger C, Leavell N-R. Marketing to America's youth: evidence from corporate documents. *Tobacco Control* 2002;11(Suppl 1):i5-i17.

6. Substance Abuse and Mental Health Services Administration. The National Survey on Drug Use and Health Report. Washington, DC: Substance Abuse and Mental Health Services Administration, Office of Applied Studies; 2007.

7. Cummings KM, Hyland A, Pechacek TF, Orlandi M, Lynn WR. Comparison of recent trends in adolescent and adult cigarette smoking behaviour and brand preferences. *Tobacco Control* 1997;6(Suppl 2):S31–S37.

8. Centers for Disease Control and Prevention. Changes in cigarette brand preferences of adolescent smokers—United States, 1989-1993. *MMWR* 1994;43(32):577–581.

9. Kaufman NJ, Castrucci BC, Mowery P, Gerlach K, Emont S, Orleans CT. Changes in adolescent cigarette-brand preference, 1989 to 1996. *American Journal of Health Behavior* 2004;28(1):54–62.

10. Institute of Medicine. *The Future of Public's Health in the 21st Century.* Washington, DC: National Academies Press; 2002.

11. California Department of Health Services. California Adult Tobacco Survey, 1997-2004. Survey instrument available at http://www.dhs.ca.gov/tobacco/html/resourceseval.htm.

12. U.S. Department of Health and Human Services. *Preventing Tobacco Use Among Young People: A Report of the Surgeon General.* Atlanta: U.S. Department of Health and Human Services, Public Health Service, Centers for Disease Control and Prevention, National Center for Chronic Disease Prevention and Health Promotion, Office on Smoking and Health; 1994.

13. Charlesworth A, Glantz SA. Tobacco and the movie industry. *Clinics in Occupational and Environmental Medicine* 2006;5(1):73–84.

14. Gilpin EA, White MM, Messer K, Pierce JP. Receptivity to tobacco advertising and promotions among young adolescents as a predictor of established smoking in young adulthood. *American Journal of Public Health* 2007;97(8):1489–1495.

15. Lovato C, Linn G, Stead LF, Best A. Impact of tobacco advertising and promotion on increasing adolescent smoking behaviours. *Cochrane Database of Systematic Reviews* 2003;(4):CD003439.

16. Federal Trade Commission. *Cigarette Report for 2004 and 2005.* Washington, DC: Federal Trade Commission; 2007.

17. Federal Trade Commission. *Smokeless Tobacco Report for the Years 2002–2005.* Washington, DC: Federal Trade Commission; 2007.

18. Wakefield M, Szczypka G, Terry-McElrath Y, Emery S, Flay B, Chaloupka F, et al. Mixed messages on tobacco: comparative exposure to public health, tobacco company- and pharmaceutical company-sponsored tobacco-related television campaigns in the United States, 1999–2003. *Addiction* 2005;100:1875–1883.

19. Pierce JP, Gilmer TP, Lee L, Gilpin EA, de Beyer J, Messer K. Tobacco industry price-subsidizing promotions may overcome the downward pressure of higher prices on initiation of regular smoking. *Health Economics* 2005;14(10):1061–1071.

20. Slater SJ, Chaloupka FJ, Wakefield M, Johnstone LD, O'Malley PM. The impact of retail cigarette marketing practices on youth smoking uptake. *Archives of Pediatric Adolescent Medicine* 2007;161:440-445.

21. Wakefield MA, Terry-McElrath YM, Chaloupka FJ, Barker DC, Slater SJ, Clark PI, et al. Tobacco industry marketing at point of purchase after the 1998 MSA billboard advertising ban. *American Journal of Public Health* 2002;92(6):937-940.

22. Farrelly MC, Healton CG, Davis KC, Messeri P, Hersey JC, Haviland ML. Getting to the truth: evaluating national tobacco countermarketing campaigns. *American Journal of Public Health* 2002;92:901–907.

23. Wakefield M, Terry-McElrath Y, Emery S, Saffer H, Chaloupka FJ, Szczypka G, et al. Effect of televised, tobacco company-funded smoking prevention advertising on youth smoking-related beliefs, intentions, and behavior. *American Journal of Public Health* 2006;96(12):2154–2160.

24. Hamilton JL. The demand for cigarettes: advertising, the health scare, and the cigarette advertising ban. *Review of Economics and Statistics* 1972;54:401–411.

25. Emery S, Wakefield MA, Terry-McElrath Y, Saffer H, Szczypka G, O'Malley PM, et al. Televised state-sponsored antitobacco advertising and youth smoking beliefs and behavior in the United States, 1999–2000. *Archives of Pediatric Adolescent Medicine* 2005;159:639-645.

26. Farrelly MC, Davis KC, Haviland L, Messeri P, Healton CG. Evidence of a dose-response relationship between "truth" antismoking ads and youth smoking prevalence. *American Journal of Public Health* 2005;95(3):425–431.

27. Centers for Disease Control and Prevention. *Designing and Implementing an Effective Tobacco Counter-Marketing Campaign.* Atlanta: U.S. Department of Health and Human Services; 2003.

28. Centers for Disease Control and Prevention. Cigarette smoking before and after an excise tax increase and anti-smoking campaign—Massachusetts, 1990–1996. *MMWR* 1996;45(44):966–970.

29. Centers for Disease Control and Prevention. Tobacco use among middle and high school students—Florida, 1998 and 1999. *MMWR* 1999;48(12):248–253.

30. Cummins SE, Hebert KK, Anderson CM, Mills JA, Zhu S-H. Reaching young adult smokers through quitlines. *American Journal of Public Health* 2007;97(8):1402–1405.

31. California Department of Health Services. California releases new data and anti-smoking ads targeting diverse populations. News Release No. 06-82, October 2, 2006. Available at http://www.dhs.ca.gov/tobacco/documents/press/PR-October-2006.pdf.

32. Centers for Disease Control and Prevention. Effect of ending an antitobacco youth campaign on adolescent susceptibility to cigarette smoking—Minnesota, 2002-2003. *MMWR* 2004;53(14):301–304.

33. Centers for Disease Control and Prevention. Decline in smoking prevalence—New York City, 2002–2006. *MMWR* 2007;56(24):604–608.

34. Flay BR. *Selling the Smokeless Society: 56 Evaluated Mass Media Programs and Campaigns Worldwide.* Washington, DC: American Public Health Association; 1987.

35. Schar E, Gutierrez K, Murphy-Hoefer R, Nelson DE. *Tobacco Use Prevention Media Campaigns: Lessons Learned from Youth in Nine Countries.* Atlanta: U.S. Department of Health and Human Services, Centers for Disease Control and Prevention, National Center for Chronic Disease Prevention and Health Promotion, Office on Smoking and Health; 2006.

36. Terry-McElrath Y, Wakefield M, Ruel E, Balch GI, Emery S, Szczypka G, et al. The effect of antismoking advertisement executional characteristics on youth comprehension, appraisal, recall, and engagement. *Journal of Health Communication* 2005;10:127–143.

37. Ibrahim JK, Glantz SA. The rise and fall of tobacco control media campaigns, 1967–2006. *American Journal of Public Health* 2007;97(8):1383–1396.

38. Centers for Disease Control and Prevention. CDCynergy, Tobacco Prevention and Control Edition. Accessible at http://apps nccd.cdc.gov/osh_pub_catalog/PublicationList.aspx (enter search term "CDCynergy").

39. Hyland A, Wakefield M, Higbee C, Szczypka G, Cummings KM. Anti-tobacco television advertising and indicators of smoking cessation in adults: a cohort study. *Health Education Research* 2006;21(2):296–302.

40. Farrelly MC, Niederdeppe J, Yarsevich J. Youth tobacco prevention mass media campaigns: past, present, and future directions. *Tobacco Control* 2003;12(Suppl 1):i35–i47.

41. Centers for Disease Control and Prevention. *Best Practices for Comprehensive Tobacco Control Programs—August 1999.* Atlanta: U.S. Department of Health and Human Services, Centers for Disease Control and Prevention, National Center for Chronic Disease Prevention and Health Promotion, Office on Smoking and Health; 1999.

42. Centers for Disease Control and Prevention. Media Campaign Resource Center Online Database. Available at http://www.cdc.gov/tobacco/media_communications/countermarketing/mcrc/index htm.

III Cessation Interventions

Justification

Interventions that increase quitting can decrease premature mortality and tobacco-related health care costs in the short-term.[1,2] Quitting by age 30 eliminates nearly all excess risk associated with smoking, and smokers who quit smoking before age 50 cut in half their risk of dying in the next 15 years.[2,3] Tobacco use screening and brief intervention by clinicians not only is a top-ranked clinical preventive service in terms of its relative health impact, effectiveness, and cost-effectiveness but also is a cost-saving measure.[4-6] Tobacco use treatment is more cost-effective than other commonly provided clinical preventive services, including mammography, colon cancer screening, Pap tests, treatment of mild to moderate hypertension, and treatment of high cholesterol.[5,7,8]

Although quitting smoking has immediate as well as long-term benefits, tobacco use is addictive. More than 40% of smokers try to quit each year, but without assistance, most will relapse.[9,10] To increase tobacco use cessation, the independent Task Force on Community Preventive Services' *Guide to Community Preventive Services* strongly recommends:[11]

- Increasing the unit price of tobacco products
- Conducting mass media education campaigns combined with other community interventions
- Providing telephone-based cessation counseling
- Reducing out-of-pocket costs for patients
- Implementing health care provider reminder systems (alone or combined with provider education)

The Public Health Service's (PHS) evidence-based clinical practice guideline on cessation states that brief advice by medical providers to quit smoking is an effective intervention.[10] More intensive interventions (individual, group, or telephone counseling) that provide social support and coaching on problem-solving skills are even more effective. FDA-approved pharmacotherapy (e.g., nicotine patch, gum, nasal spray, inhaler, and lozenge as well as non-nicotine medications such as bupropion hydrochloride and varenicline) is also proven effective in helping people quit smoking. Combining counseling and medication is most effective.

The PHS guideline stresses that health care system changes are needed (e.g., implementing a system of tobacco use screening and documentation, linking tobacco users to quitline services, and providing insurance coverage for proven treatments). Model programs in large managed care plans show that full implementation of the health care system changes, quitline services, comprehensive insurance coverage, and promotion of the services increases the use of proven treatments and decreases smoking prevalence.[12]

In 2004, the Department of Health and Human Services announced the availability of the National Network of Tobacco Cessation Quitlines, providing callers nationwide with fast and easy access to their state's quitline services through a single toll-free portal number (1-800-QUIT NOW). This service was made possible through a partnership between CDC's Office on Smoking and Health, the National Cancer Institute's Cancer Information Service, the North American Quitline Consortium, and state tobacco prevention and control programs. As of 2007, all 50 states, the District of Columbia, and five territories offer some degree of telephone-based tobacco cessation services.

State action on tobacco use treatment should include the following elements:

- Sustaining, expanding, and promoting the services available through population-based counseling and treatment programs, such as cessation quitlines
- Covering treatment for tobacco use under both public and private insurance, including individual, group, and telephone counseling and all FDA-approved medications
- Eliminating cost and other barriers to treatment for underserved populations, particularly the uninsured and populations disproportionately affected by tobacco use
- Making the health care system changes recommended by the PHS guideline

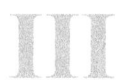

Tobacco control programs need to foster the motivation to quit through policy changes and media campaigns and promote their quitline services. The Ohio Tobacco Quit Line demonstrates the importance of promotion to generate call volume. The Quit Line received more than 100,000 calls between 2004 and 2007, reaching smokers through media campaigns, partnerships, and the offer of free nicotine replacement therapy.[13]

As a result of targeted promotion, Colorado's quitline has experienced extremely high recognition and utilization rates. During 2006–2007, 71% of Colorado smokers reported knowledge of the state quitline, and more than 9% had called for cessation assistance. This rate translates to more than 3,400 smokers enrolling each month, with a success rate at six months of 38%.[14] During 2005–2006, the Colorado tobacco control program demonstrated success in targeting cessation interventions by utilizing different spokespersons in its televised promotions. The number of African Americans calling the state's quitline nearly doubled during the phase of the campaign featuring an African American sports celebrity, compared with a promotion featuring one of his Caucasian teammates.[15]

The California Smokers' Helpline provides cessation services and culturally appropriate information in multiple languages for different audiences. Language- plus culturally-specific promotions have increased use of treatment services among tobacco users from various racial and ethnic groups.[16]

Budget

Cessation interventions should include both health care system-based interventions and population-based interventions (quitlines) that provide services to the individual smoker. System-based initiatives should ensure that all tobacco users seen in the health care system are screened for tobacco use. All tobacco users should receive advice to quit and should be offered brief or more intensive counseling services (in person or via a quitline) and FDA-approved cessation medication. Cessation quitlines are effective in increasing successful quitting and have the potential to reach large numbers of smokers. Quitlines also serve as a resource for busy health care providers, who can ask patients about their tobacco use status and then link them to quitline cessation services for counseling. Optimally, quitline counseling should be made available to all tobacco users willing to access the service.

Budget recommendations for providing health care screening and brief interventions are based on the 1999 funding formula, adjusted for changes in state population and inflation. The recommended level of investment for telephone-based cessation services has been updated to reflect new evidence regarding attainable rates of quitline usage and limited provision of no-cost or low-cost over-the-counter nicotine replacement therapy (NRT). With sufficient promotion and clinician referral, and with NRT made more easily available, a state quitline could serve 8% of tobacco users aged 18 years and older. Budget estimates assumed approximately 75% of callers (6% of a state's tobacco users) would seek counseling services, and of those, approximately 85% would accept NRT if it is offered. State experience suggests that programs should offer two weeks of free NRT to all callers receiving counseling and at least four weeks for callers who are uninsured or who receive publicly financed insurance.

The funding range for Cessation Interventions allows for variability in the percentage of callers who receive counseling (from 2% to 10%) and the amount of NRT provided. The funding model includes a minimum of two weeks of NRT for all callers enrolled in counseling anticipated to accept NRT, ranging up to an eight-week course for those who are uninsured or receiving publicly financed insurance. However, it is expected that states will work with Medicaid and private insurers to ensure comprehensive insurance coverage of tobacco use treatment by all insurers. States may also be able to lower implementation costs by engaging in cost-sharing partnerships with Medicaid and health insurance providers for the provision of NRT and other services. Negotiating volume discounts can also decrease the cost of providing NRT.

III Cessation Interventions

Core Resources

Zaza S, Briss PA, Harris KW, editors. *The Guide to Community Preventive Services: What Works to Promote Health?* New York: Oxford University Press; 2005. Available at http://www.thecommunityguide.org/tobacco/default htm.

Fiore MC, Bailey WC, Cohen SJ, Dorfman SF, Goldstein MG, Gritz ER, et al. *Treating Tobacco Use and Dependence. Clinical Practice Guideline.* Rockville, MD: U.S. Department of Health and Human Services, Public Health Service; 2000. Available at http://www.surgeongeneral.gov/tobacco/treating_tobacco_use.pdf.

US Department of Health and Human Services. *Reducing Tobacco Use: A Report of the Surgeon General.* Atlanta: U.S. Department of Health and Human Services, Centers for Disease Control and Prevention, National Center for Chronic Disease Prevention and Health Promotion, Office on Smoking and Health; 2000. Available at http://www.cdc.gov/tobacco/data_statistics/sgr/sgr_2000/index.htm.

Centers for Disease Control and Prevention. *Coverage for Tobacco Use Cessation Treatments.* Atlanta: U.S. Department of Health and Human Services, Centers for Disease Control and Prevention, National Center for Chronic Disease Prevention and Health Promotion, Office on Smoking and Health; 2003. Available at http://www.cdc.gov/tobacco/quit_smoking/cessation/coverage/index htm.

Centers for Disease Control and Prevention. *A Practical Guide to Working with Health-Care Systems on Tobacco-Use Treatment.* Atlanta: U.S. Department of Health and Human Services, Centers for Disease Control and Prevention, National Center for Chronic Disease Prevention and Health Promotion, Office on Smoking and Health; 2006. Available at http://www.cdc.gov/tobacco/quit_smoking/cessation/practicalguide htm.

Centers for Disease Control and Prevention. *Telephone Quitlines: A Resource for Development, Implementation, and Evaluation.* Atlanta: U.S. Department of Health and Human Services, Centers for Disease Control and Prevention, National Center for Chronic Disease Prevention and Health Promotion, Office on Smoking and Health; 2004. Available at http://www.cdc.gov/tobacco/quit_smoking/cessation/quitlines/index htm.

North American Quitline Consortium. *Quitline Operations: A Practical Guide to Promising Approaches.* Phoenix, AZ: North American Quitline Consortium; 2005. Available at http://www.naquitline.org/pdfs/quitline_approaches.pdf.

National Cancer Institute. Smokefree.gov. Available at www.smokefree.gov.

North American Quitline Consortium. Available at http://www.naquitline.org/welcome.asp.

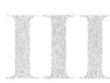

References

1. Curry SJ, Grothaus LC, McAfee, T, Pabiniak C. Use and cost effectiveness of smoking-cessation services under four insurance plans in a health maintenance organization. *New England Journal of Medicine* 1998;339(10):673–679.

2. U.S. Department of Health and Human Services. *The Health Benefits of Smoking Cessation: A Report of the Surgeon General.* Atlanta: U.S. Department of Health and Human Services, Centers for Disease Control and Prevention; 1990. DHHS Publication No. (CDC)90–8416.

3. Doll R, Peto R, Boreham J, Sutherland I. Mortality in relation to smoking: 50 years' observations on male British doctors. *British Medical Journal* 2004;328:1519–1527.

4. Solberg LI, Maciosek MV, Edwards NM, Khanchandani HS, Goodman MJ. Repeated tobacco use screening and intervention in clinical practice: health impact and cost effectiveness. *American Journal of Preventive Medicine* 2006;31(1):62–71.

5. Maciosek MV, Coffield AB, Edwards NM, Flottemesch TJ, Goodman MJ, Solberg LI. Priorities among effective clinical preventive services: results of a systematic review and analysis. *American Journal of Preventive Medicine* 2006;31(1)52–61.

6. Marks JS, Koplan JP, Hogue CJ, Dalmat ME. A cost-benefit/cost-effectiveness analysis of smoking cessation for pregnant women. *American Journal of Preventive Medicine* 1990;6(5):282-289.

7. Cummings SR, Rubin SM, Oster G. The cost-effectiveness of counseling smokers to quit. *JAMA* 1989;261:75–79.

8. Tsevat J. Impact and cost-effectiveness of smoking interventions. *American Journal of Medicine* 1992;93:43S–47S.

9. Centers for Disease Control and Prevention. Tobacco use among adults—United States, 2005. *MMWR* 2006;55(42):1145-1148.

10. Fiore MC, Bailey WC, Cohen SJ, Dorfman SF, Goldstein MG, Gritz ER, et al. *Treating Tobacco Use and Dependence. Clinical Practice Guideline.* Rockville, MD: U.S. Department of Health and Human Services, Public Health Service; 2000.

11. Zaza S, Briss PA, Harris KW, editors. *The Guide to Community Preventive Services: What Works to Promote Health?* New York: Oxford University Press; 2005.

12. Thompson RS, Taplin SH, McAfee TA, Mandelson MT, Smith AE. Primary and secondary prevention services in clinical practice. Twenty years' experience in development, implementation, and evaluation. *JAMA* 1995;273(14):1130–1135.

13. Ohio Tobacco Prevention Foundation. Information for Policymakers. Available at http://www.otpf.org/audience/audience.aspx?id =4930&Audience=Policymakers.

14. National Jewish Medical and Research Center. *Tobacco Cessation Outcome Results for the State Tobacco Educational and Prevention Partnership (STEPP)—August 2007.* Denver, CO: National Jewish Medical and Research Center; 2007.

15. SHiFT Incorporated. *STEPP/Adult Cessation Annual Project Report: Colorado QuitLine TV Campaign with John Lynch/Kyle Johnson.* Denver, CO: SHiFT Incorporated; 2007.

16. California Department of Health Services. California releases new data and anti-smoking ads targeting diverse populations. News Release No. 06-82, October 2, 2006. Available at http://www.dhs.ca.gov/tobacco/documents/ press/PR-October-2006.pdf.

IV Surveillance and Evaluation

Justification

Publicly financed programs need to have accountability and demonstrate effectiveness. A comprehensive tobacco control program must have a system of surveillance and evaluation that can monitor and document short-term, intermediate, and long-term intervention outcomes in the population to inform program and policy direction, as well as to ensure accountability to those with fiscal oversight.

State surveillance is the process of monitoring tobacco-related attitudes, behaviors, and health outcomes at regular intervals of time. Statewide surveillance should monitor the achievement of the four primary program goals: 1) preventing initiation of tobacco use among youth and young adults, 2) promoting quitting among adults and youth, 3) eliminating exposure to secondhand smoke, and 4) identifying and eliminating tobacco-related disparities among population groups. Participation in national surveillance systems (e.g., the Behavioral Risk Factor Surveillance System, Youth Risk Behavior Surveillance System, and Pregnancy Risk Assessment Monitoring System) enables a state to compare some of its long-term tobacco measures to those of other states.[1-3] These data can be used to compare a state's program impact and outcomes with national trends. In addition, states have enhanced these national systems by adding state-specific questions and modules, increasing sample sizes to capture local and specific population data, and modifying sampling procedures to provide more data on intermediate performance objectives.

Specific systems to collect evaluation data are also needed. Process and outcome evaluation activities should be ongoing and should be used to assess individual program activities and to guide program improvement. Program evaluation efforts should build on and complement data collection by linking statewide and local program efforts to monitor progress toward program objectives. Additionally, evaluation can provide valuable data on the relative effectiveness of specific innovative program activities. States can contribute to the literature on best practices by publishing their evaluation results.

Flexible survey instruments for use in program evaluation include the Youth Tobacco Survey and Adult Tobacco Survey.[4] These surveys maintain some standard "core" components, but they also allow states to include questions to evaluate current program activity. Both surveys provide state-level data that can be compared with those from other states and include data on many key outcome indicators for evaluation of comprehensive tobacco control programs. For both evaluation tools, estimates can be obtained at the regional, county, or city level, with appropriate sampling. State-level data also can be compared with national data.

Program evaluation requires that a wide range of short-term and intermediate indicators of program effectiveness be measured, including policy changes, changes in social norms, and exposure of individuals and communities to statewide and local program efforts. Evaluation efforts should also include counter-marketing surveillance to track new products and examine the impact of pro-tobacco influences, including the actual cost of cigarettes, free samples, advertising, promotions, media coverage, and events that glamorize tobacco use. In addition, evaluation requires collection of data such as information from the quitline Minimal Data Set, legislative tracking, vital statistics, Synar compliance data, observational studies, Nielsen data, opinion surveys, air quality studies, media evaluation, or program monitoring data (e.g., tracking alignment of local program efforts with statewide priorities).

Evaluation planning should be integrated with program planning. A comprehensive state tobacco control plan—with well-defined goals; objectives; and short-term, intermediate, and long-term indicators—requires appropriate surveillance and evaluation data systems. Collection of baseline data related to each objective and outcome indicator is critical to ensuring that program-related effects can be clearly measured. For this reason, surveillance and evaluation systems must have first priority in the planning process.

CDC's Office on Smoking and Health developed *Introduction to Program Evaluation for Comprehensive Tobacco Control Programs,* a "how-to" guide for planning and implementing evaluation activities.[5] *Key Outcome Indicators for Evaluating Comprehensive*

Surveillance and Evaluation IV

Tobacco Control Programs is a companion piece that provides information on selecting evidence-based indicators and linking them to program outcomes.[6] *Surveillance and Data Resources for Comprehensive Tobacco Control Programs* provides a summary of the tobacco-related measures, sampling frame, and methodology for many national and state surveys and tools for use in conducting surveillance and evaluation efforts.[7]

In order to develop effective interventions and to monitor progress, most states need more information on populations disproportionately affected by tobacco use. If standard data collections do not provide adequate data to characterize health disparities related to tobacco use, additional data collection systems or approaches may be needed (e.g., snowball sampling techniques with disparate groups). For instance, in 2004 California conducted population-specific tobacco use surveys to identify tobacco-related knowledge, attitudes, and behaviors among the state's Asian Indian; Korean American; Chinese American; active duty military; and Lesbian, Gay, Bisexual, and Transgender adult populations. Similarly, several major North American tribes have conducted tobacco use surveys both in schools and among adults to collect more detailed data on their populations to inform program development. For more information on identifying and eliminating tobacco-related disparities, see Appendix D. Some available tools for surveillance and evaluation include:

- The Youth Tobacco Survey (YTS) is a school-based state-level survey of young people in grades 6 through 12. Core questions assess students' knowledge, attitudes, and behaviors related to tobacco use and exposure to secondhand smoke, as well as their exposure to prevention curricula, community programs, and media messages aimed at preventing and reducing youth tobacco use. YTS also collects information on the effectiveness of enforcement measures. The Adult Tobacco Survey is a telephone survey of adults aged 18 years and older. Core questions assess adults' knowledge, attitudes, and behaviors related to tobacco use, exposure to secondhand smoke, use of cessation assistance, and their awareness of and support for evidence-based policy interventions.

- The State Tobacco Activities Tracking and Evaluation (STATE) System is an online data warehouse that includes epidemiologic data on many long-term key outcome indicators, as well as economic data and tobacco-related state legislation.[8]

- NCI and CDC added tobacco modules to the Current Population Surveys in 1992–1993, 1995–1996, 1998–1999, 2002–2003, and 2006–2007.[9] These modules provide state-specific estimates on factors such as smoking prevalence, quit attempts, exposure to secondhand smoke at home and work, workplace policies, and cessation counseling by physicians and dentists among adults aged 18 years and older.

- The quitline Minimum Data Set identifies a recommended set of indicators collected in a consistent manner to facilitate performance monitoring and make comparisons possible, while not imposing undue burdens on quitlines.[10]

- In conducting more detailed evaluation of major program elements, particularly media campaigns, several states have conducted periodic special statewide surveys of adults and young people. Examples of methodology for state-specific surveys are described in California's evaluation reports.[11]

CDC's *Evidence of Effectiveness: A Summary of State Tobacco Control Program Evaluation Literature* provides examples of state tobacco control program evaluations and their outcomes, as well as references to scientific literature by major findings (e.g., heart disease mortality, youth smoking prevalence/initiation, or per capita consumption).[12]

Additional resources will soon be available, including CDC's *Introduction to Process Evaluation in Tobacco Use Prevention and Control*, which provides guidance to states about how to evaluate inputs, activities, and outputs of a tobacco control logic model; *Tobacco Counter-Marketing Paid Media Evaluation Manual*, which outlines various ways of evaluating state media campaigns; and a National Cancer Institute (NCI) media monograph with information about the relevant theories behind media campaigns, descriptions of effective campaigns, and information on campaign evaluation.

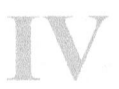 **Surveillance and Evaluation**

Budget

All federally funded tobacco prevention and control programs are expected to engage in strategic surveillance and program evaluation activities. State health departments currently manage most tobacco surveillance systems. Many states work in conjunction with universities to implement and coordinate surveillance, evaluation, and research activities. Standard practice dictates that about 10% of total annual program funds be allocated for surveillance and evaluation.[13,14] Additional resources beyond 10% of program funds may be required for development of effective local capacity for evaluation and for conducting detailed evaluation of specific media, cessation, and community interventions. For example, obtaining population-representative data for local jurisdictions (e.g., counties) or conducting cohort studies to assess the effectiveness of media campaigns can be resource intensive. Thus, health departments must be able to expand their evaluation resources as needed.

Reaching the national goal of eliminating health disparities related to tobacco use will necessitate improved collection and use of standardized data to correctly identify disparities in both health outcomes and efficacy of interventions among various population groups.[15] Additional data collection mechanisms and standardized systems may be needed to better characterize health disparities related to tobacco use and measure progress toward eliminating these disparities.

Experience has shown that evaluation efforts can be used both for statewide surveillance and evaluation systems and for increased technical capacity of local programs to perform process and outcome evaluation activities. For example, in California, every grantee must spend 10% of its budget on evaluating its own activities. To aid this activity, the California Tobacco Control Program publishes a directory of evaluators who can consult with their local programs and conduct local program evaluations and funds a local program evaluation center that provides technical assistance to its contractors.[11]

Core Resources

MacDonald G, Starr G, Schooley M, Yee SL, Klimowski K, Turner K. *Introduction to Program Evaluation for Comprehensive Tobacco Control Programs.* Atlanta: Centers for Disease Control and Prevention; 2001. Available at http://www.cdc.gov/tobacco/tobacco_control_programs/surveillance_evaluation/evaluation_manual/index htm.

Yee SL, Schooley M. *Surveillance and Evaluation Data Resources for Comprehensive Tobacco Control Programs.* Atlanta: Centers for Disease Control and Prevention; 2001. Available at http://www.cdc.gov/tobacco/tobacco_control_programs/surveillance_evaluation/surveillance_manual/index.htm.

Starr G, Rogers T, Schooley M, Porter S, Wiesen E, Jamison N. *Key Outcome Indicators for Evaluating Comprehensive Tobacco Control Programs.* Atlanta: Centers for Disease Control and Prevention; 2005. Available at http://www.cdc.gov/tobacco/tobacco_control_programs/surveillance_evaluation/key_outcome/index.htm.

Centers for Disease Control and Prevention. *Sustaining State Programs for Tobacco Control: Data Highlights 2006.* Atlanta: Centers for Disease Control and Prevention, National Center for Chronic Disease Prevention and Health Promotion, Office on Smoking and Health; 2006. Available at http://www.cdc.gov/tobacco/data_statistics/state_data/data_highlights/2006/index.htm.

Kuiper NM, Nelson DE, Schooley M. *Evidence of Effectiveness: A Summary of State Tobacco Control Program Evaluation Literature.* Atlanta: Centers for Disease Control and Prevention, National Center for Chronic Disease Prevention and Health Promotion, Office on Smoking and Health; 2005. Available at http://www.cdc.gov/tobacco/tobacco_control_programs/stateandcommunity/sustainingstates/00_pdfs/lit_Review.pdf.

Centers for Disease Control and Prevention. *Introduction to Process Evaluation in Tobacco Use Prevention and Control.* Atlanta: Centers for Disease Control and Prevention. In press.

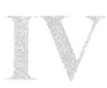
Murphy-Hoefer R, Porter S, Nierderdeppe J, Farrelly M, Sly D, Yarsevich J. *Introduction to Countermarketing Evaluation for Comprehensive Tobacco Control Programs.* Atlanta: Centers for Disease Control and Prevention. In press.

North American Quitline Consortium. Quitline Minimal Data Set. Available at http://www.naquitline.org/index.asp?dbid=2&dbsection=research.

Centers for Disease Control and Prevention. State Tobacco Activities Tracking and Evaluation (STATE) System. Available at http://apps.nccd.cdc.gov/statesystem.

Centers for Disease Control and Prevention. Smoking & Tobacco Use website. Available at www.cdc.gov/tobacco.

References

1. Centers for Disease Control and Prevention. Behavioral Risk Factor Surveillance System (BRFSS). Available at http://www.cdc.gov/brfss/.
2. Centers for Disease Control and Prevention. Youth Risk Behavior Surveillance System (YRBSS). Available at http://www.cdc.gov/healthyyouth/yrbs/index.htm.
3. Centers for Disease Control and Prevention. Pregnancy Risk Assessment Monitoring System (PRAMS). Available at http://www.cdc.gov/PRAMS/.
4. Centers for Disease Control and Prevention. Youth Tobacco Survey (YTS). Available at http://www.cdc.gov/tobacco/data_statistics/surveys/YTS/index htm.
5. MacDonald G, Starr G, Schooley M, Yee SL, Klimowski K, Turner K. *Introduction to Program Evaluation for Comprehensive Tobacco Control Programs.* Atlanta: Centers for Disease Control and Prevention; 2001.
6. Starr G, Rogers T, Schooley M, Porter S, Wiesen E, Jamison N. *Key Outcome Indicators for Evaluating Comprehensive Tobacco Control Programs.* Atlanta: Centers for Disease Control and Prevention; 2005.
7. Yee SL, Schooley M. *Surveillance and Evaluation Data Resources for Comprehensive Tobacco Control Programs.* Atlanta: Centers for Disease Control and Prevention; 2001.
8. Centers for Disease Control and Prevention. State Tobacco Activities Tracking and Evaluation (STATE) System. Available at http://apps.nccd.cdc.gov/statesystem.
9. National Cancer Institute. Tobacco Use Supplement to the Current Population Survey (TUS-CPS). Available at http://riskfactor.cancer.gov/studies/tus-cps/.
10. North American Quitline Consortium. Quitline Minimal Data Set. Available at http://www naquitline.org/index.asp?dbid=2&dbsection=research.
11. California Department of Health Services, Tobacco Control Section, Evaluation Resources. Available at http://www.dhs.ca.gov/tobacco/html/resourceseval.htm#evaluation.
12. Kuiper NM, Nelson DE, Schooley M. *Evidence of Effectiveness: A Summary of State Tobacco Control Program Evaluation Literature.* Atlanta: Centers for Disease Control and Prevention, National Center for Chronic Disease Prevention and Health Promotion, Office on Smoking and Health; 2005.
13. World Health Organization European Working Group on Health Promotion Evaluation. *Health Promotion Evaluation: Recommendations to Policy-makers: Report of the WHO European Working Group on Health Promotion Evaluation.* Copenhagen, Denmark: World Health Organization, Regional Office for Europe; 1998.
14. Centers for Disease Control and Prevention. *Best Practices for Comprehensive Tobacco Control Programs—August 1999.* Atlanta: U.S. Department of Health and Human Services, Centers for Disease Control and Prevention, National Center for Chronic Disease Prevention and Health Promotion, Office on Smoking and Health; 1999.
15. U.S. Department of Health and Human Services. *Reducing Tobacco Use: A Report of the Surgeon General.* Atlanta: U.S. Department of Health and Human Services, Centers for Disease Control and Prevention, National Center for Chronic Disease Prevention and Health Promotion, Office on Smoking and Health; 2000.

V Administration and Management

Justification

Effective tobacco prevention and control programs require substantial funding to implement, thus making the need for good fiscal management and accountability critical. Internal capacity within a state health department is essential for program sustainability, efficacy, and efficiency.[1-3] Sufficient capacity enables programs to plan their strategic efforts, provide strong leadership, and foster collaboration among the state and local tobacco control community. An adequate number of skilled staff is also necessary to provide or facilitate program oversight, technical assistance, and training.

State experience has shown the importance of having all of the program's components coordinated and working together. New York, Oklahoma, and Indiana structured their programs in such a way that Administration and Management served as an umbrella category, providing oversight for all of their tobacco prevention and control interventions.[4] The ASSIST evaluation demonstrates the importance of state health department infrastructure, experienced staff, and strong partnerships.[5]

Program management and coordination present a challenge in that a comprehensive program involves multiple state agencies (e.g., public health, education, and law enforcement) and levels of local government; other public health programs; and numerous health-related voluntary organizations, coalitions, and community groups. Furthermore, coordinating and integrating major statewide programs (e.g., counter-marketing campaigns, telephone quitlines) with local program efforts requires adequate staffing and efficient communication systems.

Because it takes time and resources to establish the capacity needed to implement effective interventions, it is critical to sustain an established infrastructure. Once a strong foundation is in place, a cumulative effect of funding on program efficacy is evident. Research shows that the longer states invest in such programs, the greater and faster the impact.[6]

Administration and management activities include the following:

- Engaging in strategic planning to guide program efforts and resources to accomplish their goals
- Recruiting and developing qualified and diverse technical, program, and administrative staff
- Awarding and monitoring program contracts and grants, coordinating implementation across program areas, and assessing grantee program performance
- Developing and maintaining a real-time fiscal management system that tracks allocations and expenditure of funds
- Increasing capacity at the local level by providing ongoing training and technical assistance
- Creating an effective communication system internally, across chronic disease programs, and with local coalitions and partners
- Educating the public and decision makers on the health effects of tobacco and evidence-based effective program and policy interventions

Budget

Best practices dictate that about 5% of total annual program funds be allocated to state program Administration and Management. These funds should be used to ensure collaboration and coordination among public health program managers, policy makers, and other state agencies. Because of the importance of maintaining an infrastructure and the capacity to provide guidance, technical assistance, and coordination among programs and networks, 5% of the CDC-recommended level of investment for interventions remains the suggested budgeting target for administration and management activities, even if actual program funding is below the CDC-recommended amount.

Core Resources

California Department of Health Services. *A Model for Change: The California Experience in Tobacco Control.* Sacramento: California Department of Health Services; 1998.

California Department of Health Services. *California Tobacco Control Update 2006: The Social Norm Change Approach.* Sacramento: California Department of Health Services; 2006.

Center for Tobacco Policy Research. *Project LEaP: Linking Evaluation and Practice in Tobacco Control.* Saint Louis, MO: Saint Louis University School of Public Health; 2005. Available at http://ctpr.slu.edu/leap.php#phase1.

National Cancer Institute. *Evaluating ASSIST: A Blueprint for Understanding State-Level Tobacco Control.* Tobacco Control Monograph No. 17. Bethesda, MD: U.S. Department of Health and Human Services, National Institutes of Health, National Cancer Institute; 2006. NIH Pub. No. 06-6058. Available at http://cancercontrol.cancer.gov/tcrb/monographs/17/index html.

U.S. Department of Health and Human Services. *Reducing Tobacco Use: A Report of the Surgeon General.* Atlanta: U.S. Department of Health and Human Services, Centers for Disease Control and Prevention, National Center for Chronic Disease Prevention and Health Promotion, Office on Smoking and Health; 2000. Available at http://www.cdc.gov/tobacco/data_statistics/sgr/sgr_2000/index htm.

Zaza S, Briss PA, Harris KW, editors. *The Guide to Community Preventive Services: What Works to Promote Health?* New York: Oxford University Press; 2005. Available at http://www.thecommunityguide.org/tobacco/default htm.

References

1. Center for Tobacco Policy Research. *Project LEaP: Linking Evaluation and Practice in Tobacco Control.* Saint Louis, MO: Saint Louis University School of Public Health; 2005.

2. Nelson DE, Reynolds JH, Luke DA, Mueller NB, Eischen MH, Jordan J, et al. Successfully maintaining program funding during trying times: lessons from tobacco control programs in five states. *Journal of Public Health Management & Practice.* In press.

3. National Cancer Institute. *ASSIST: Shaping the Future of Tobacco Prevention and Control.* Tobacco Control Monograph No. 16. Bethesda, MD: U.S. Department of Health and Human Services, National Institutes of Health, National Cancer Institute; 2005. NIH Pub No. 05-5645.

4. Mueller NB, Luke DA, Herbers SH, Montgomery TP. The best practices: use of the guidelines by ten state tobacco control programs. *American Journal of Preventive Medicine* 2006;31(4):300–306.

5. National Cancer Institute. *Evaluating ASSIST: A Blueprint for Understanding State-Level Tobacco Control.* Tobacco Control Monograph No. 17. Bethesda, MD: U.S. Department of Health and Human Services, National Institutes of Health, National Cancer Institute; 2006. NIH Pub. No. 06-6058.

6. Farrelly MC, Pechacek TP, Chaloupka FJ. The impact of tobacco control program expenditures on aggregate cigarette sales: 1981–2000. *Journal of Health Economics* 2003;22(5):843–859.

Section B

CDC Recommended Annual Per Capita Funding Levels for State Programs, 2007

State	Total Recommended Program Costs			State and Community Interventions			Health Communication Interventions		
	Recommended	Lower	Upper	Recommended	Lower	Upper	Recommended	Lower	Upper
United States	12.34	8.43	18.27	4.88	3.99	6.75	2.36	1.30	3.90
Alabama	12.31	8.75	19.38	5.04	4.07	6.87	1.69	1.30	3.90
Alaska	16.11	11.72	23.96	7.93	6.69	10.81	2.13	1.30	3.90
Arizona	11.03	8.30	17.94	4.70	4.00	6.77	1.64	1.30	3.90
Arkansas	12.91	9.04	19.87	5.43	4.30	7.22	1.78	1.30	3.90
California	12.12	7.85	16.75	4.68	3.78	6.44	3.02	1.30	3.90
Colorado	11.46	8.37	17.85	4.89	4.03	6.81	1.81	1.30	3.90
Connecticut	12.54	8.61	18.06	5.09	4.26	7.16	2.63	1.30	3.90
Delaware	16.32	10.80	22.07	6.52	5.92	9.66	3.90	1.30	3.90
District of Columbia	18.02	11.83	23.37	8.27	6.92	11.15	3.90	1.30	3.90
Florida	11.66	8.25	18.36	4.35	3.69	6.30	2.00	1.30	3.90
Georgia	12.44	8.26	18.07	4.74	3.87	6.57	2.62	1.30	3.90
Hawaii	11.80	9.64	19.62	5.55	5.12	8.44	1.46	1.30	3.90
Idaho	11.50	9.35	19.12	5.36	5.00	8.27	1.61	1.30	3.90
Illinois	12.23	8.28	18.12	4.93	3.83	6.52	2.14	1.30	3.90
Indiana	12.46	8.66	19.19	4.99	3.96	6.71	1.83	1.30	3.90
Iowa	12.29	8.92	19.10	5.37	4.29	7.21	1.60	1.30	3.90
Kansas	11.60	8.87	18.81	5.31	4.37	7.32	1.30	1.30	3.90
Kentucky	13.59	9.13	20.71	5.50	4.09	6.91	1.65	1.30	3.90
Louisiana	12.46	8.90	19.63	5.31	4.22	7.10	1.59	1.30	3.90
Maine	13.92	9.82	20.74	5.87	5.04	8.34	2.41	1.30	3.90
Maryland	11.26	8.35	17.77	4.38	4.01	6.79	2.17	1.30	3.90
Massachusetts	13.98	8.29	17.79	4.92	3.92	6.65	3.90	1.30	3.90
Michigan	11.99	8.49	18.70	4.94	3.89	6.60	1.66	1.30	3.90
Minnesota	11.31	8.40	17.81	4.77	4.02	6.80	1.77	1.30	3.90
Mississippi	13.47	9.13	20.34	5.44	4.35	7.30	2.13	1.30	3.90
Missouri	12.52	8.64	19.06	4.95	3.97	6.72	1.99	1.30	3.90
Montana	14.79	10.31	21.00	6.71	5.62	9.21	2.69	1.30	3.90
Nebraska	12.20	9.23	19.18	5.29	4.76	7.92	2.00	1.30	3.90
Nevada	13.08	9.04	19.53	5.42	4.41	7.39	2.18	1.30	3.90
New Hampshire	14.58	9.72	19.88	5.37	5.11	8.44	3.90	1.30	3.90
New Jersey	13.75	8.27	17.70	4.76	3.92	6.65	3.90	1.30	3.90
New Mexico	11.95	9.15	19.51	5.55	4.62	7.70	1.33	1.30	3.90
New York	13.15	8.03	17.57	4.65	3.69	6.31	3.42	1.30	3.90
North Carolina	12.06	8.40	18.63	4.84	3.82	6.50	1.83	1.30	3.90
North Dakota	14.67	11.49	22.69	7.37	6.61	10.68	1.86	1.30	3.90
Ohio	12.64	8.42	18.61	5.12	3.82	6.50	2.02	1.30	3.90
Oklahoma	12.54	8.98	20.02	5.38	4.19	7.06	1.34	1.30	3.90
Oregon	11.60	8.50	18.25	4.80	4.07	6.88	1.88	1.30	3.90
Pennsylvania	12.49	8.35	18.33	4.49	3.76	6.40	2.57	1.30	3.90
Rhode Island	14.21	10.15	20.89	6.28	5.45	8.95	2.53	1.30	3.90
South Carolina	14.39	8.73	19.24	4.74	4.09	6.91	3.90	1.30	3.90
South Dakota	14.44	10.87	21.88	7.05	6.08	9.90	1.97	1.30	3.90
Tennessee	11.89	8.55	19.04	4.67	3.92	6.66	1.75	1.30	3.90
Texas	11.31	8.06	17.48	4.85	3.84	6.52	1.83	1.30	3.90
Utah	9.23	8.31	16.48	4.55	4.55	7.60	1.44	1.30	3.90
Vermont	16.75	11.56	22.85	7.39	6.71	10.84	3.74	1.30	3.90
Virginia	13.50	8.30	17.93	4.37	3.87	6.58	3.90	1.30	3.90
Washington	10.50	8.20	17.48	4.51	3.91	6.64	1.44	1.30	3.90
West Virginia	15.33	9.64	21.25	5.74	4.61	7.68	3.13	1.30	3.90
Wisconsin	11.59	8.55	18.54	4.97	4.01	6.79	1.45	1.30	3.90
Wyoming	17.38	12.44	24.58	8.50	7.35	11.80	2.84	1.30	3.90

CDC Recommended Annual Per Capita Funding Levels for State Programs, 2007

Cessation Interventions			Surveillance and Evaluation			Administration and Management			2006 Population Estimate (millions)
Recommended	Lower	Upper	Recommended	Lower	Upper	Recommended	Lower	Upper	
3.49	2.04	5.24	1.07	0.73	1.59	0.54	0.37	0.79	299.403
3.97	2.24	6.08	1.07	0.76	1.69	0.54	0.38	0.84	4.599
3.95	2.20	6.13	1.40	1.02	2.08	0.70	0.51	1.04	0.670
3.25	1.92	4.93	0.96	0.72	1.56	0.48	0.36	0.78	6.166
4.02	2.26	6.16	1.12	0.79	1.73	0.56	0.39	0.86	2.811
2.84	1.75	4.22	1.05	0.68	1.46	0.53	0.34	0.73	36.458
3.26	1.95	4.81	1.00	0.73	1.55	0.50	0.36	0.78	4.753
3.18	1.93	4.64	1.09	0.75	1.57	0.55	0.37	0.79	3.505
3.77	2.17	5.63	1.42	0.94	1.92	0.71	0.47	0.96	0.853
3.50	2.07	5.27	1.57	1.03	2.03	0.78	0.51	1.02	0.582
3.79	2.18	5.76	1.01	0.72	1.60	0.51	0.36	0.80	18.090
3.46	2.01	5.24	1.08	0.72	1.57	0.54	0.36	0.79	9.364
3.25	1.96	4.72	1.03	0.84	1.71	0.51	0.42	0.85	1.285
3.03	1.83	4.46	1.00	0.81	1.66	0.50	0.41	0.83	1.466
3.57	2.07	5.33	1.06	0.72	1.58	0.53	0.36	0.79	12.832
4.02	2.27	6.08	1.08	0.75	1.67	0.54	0.38	0.83	6.314
3.72	2.16	5.50	1.07	0.78	1.66	0.53	0.39	0.83	2.982
3.48	2.04	5.13	1.01	0.77	1.64	0.50	0.39	0.82	2.764
4.67	2.55	7.20	1.18	0.79	1.80	0.59	0.40	0.90	4.206
3.94	2.22	6.07	1.08	0.77	1.71	0.54	0.39	0.85	4.288
3.82	2.20	5.80	1.21	0.85	1.80	0.61	0.43	0.90	1.322
3.24	1.95	4.76	0.98	0.73	1.55	0.49	0.36	0.77	5.616
3.33	1.99	4.92	1.22	0.72	1.55	0.61	0.36	0.77	6.437
3.83	2.19	5.76	1.04	0.74	1.63	0.52	0.37	0.81	10.096
3.30	1.98	4.79	0.98	0.73	1.55	0.49	0.37	0.77	5.167
4.14	2.29	6.49	1.17	0.79	1.77	0.59	0.40	0.88	2.911
3.95	2.24	5.95	1.09	0.75	1.66	0.54	0.38	0.83	5.843
3.46	2.04	5.15	1.29	0.90	1.83	0.64	0.45	0.91	0.945
3.32	1.97	4.86	1.06	0.80	1.67	0.53	0.40	0.83	1.768
3.77	2.15	5.69	1.14	0.79	1.70	0.57	0.39	0.85	2.496
3.41	2.04	4.95	1.27	0.85	1.73	0.63	0.42	0.86	1.315
3.29	1.97	4.84	1.20	0.72	1.54	0.60	0.36	0.77	8.725
3.51	2.03	5.36	1.04	0.80	1.70	0.52	0.40	0.85	1.955
3.37	1.99	5.07	1.14	0.70	1.53	0.57	0.35	0.76	19.306
3.82	2.18	5.80	1.05	0.73	1.62	0.52	0.37	0.81	8.857
3.52	2.08	5.15	1.28	1.00	1.97	0.64	0.50	0.99	0.636
3.85	2.20	5.78	1.10	0.73	1.62	0.55	0.37	0.81	11.478
4.18	2.32	6.45	1.09	0.78	1.74	0.55	0.39	0.87	3.579
3.41	2.02	5.09	1.01	0.74	1.59	0.50	0.37	0.79	3.701
3.80	2.20	5.64	1.09	0.73	1.59	0.54	0.36	0.80	12.441
3.54	2.08	5.31	1.24	0.88	1.82	0.62	0.44	0.91	1.068
3.87	2.20	5.92	1.25	0.76	1.67	0.63	0.38	0.84	4.321
3.53	2.07	5.23	1.26	0.95	1.90	0.63	0.47	0.95	0.782
3.92	2.22	5.99	1.03	0.74	1.66	0.52	0.37	0.83	6.039
3.16	1.87	4.78	0.98	0.70	1.52	0.49	0.35	0.76	23.508
2.04	1.38	2.83	0.80	0.72	1.43	0.40	0.36	0.72	2.550
3.43	2.04	5.13	1.46	1.01	1.99	0.73	0.50	0.99	0.624
3.47	2.05	5.11	1.17	0.72	1.56	0.59	0.36	0.78	7.643
3.18	1.92	4.66	0.91	0.71	1.52	0.46	0.36	0.76	6.396
4.46	2.47	6.90	1.33	0.84	1.85	0.67	0.42	0.92	1.818
3.66	2.13	5.43	1.01	0.74	1.61	0.50	0.37	0.81	5.557
3.77	2.17	5.67	1.51	1.08	2.14	0.76	0.54	1.07	0.515

CDC Recommended Annual Total Funding Levels for State Programs, 2007

State	Total Recommended Program Costs			State and Community Interventions			Health Communication Interventions		
	Recommended (millions)	Lower (millions)	Upper (millions)	Recommended (millions)	Lower (millions)	Upper (millions)	Recommended (millions)	Lower (millions)	Upper (millions)
United States	3,696.6	2,524.0	5,473.8	1,461.3	1,194.1	2,022.4	706.7	389.4	1,167.6
Alabama	56.7	40.3	89.2	23.2	18.7	31.6	7.8	6.0	17.9
Alaska	10.7	7.9	16.0	5.3	4.5	7.2	1.4	0.9	2.6
Arizona	68.1	51.2	110.5	29.0	24.7	41.7	10.1	8.0	24.0
Arkansas	36.4	25.5	55.9	15.3	12.1	20.3	5.0	3.7	11.0
California	441.9	286.2	610.4	170.6	137.8	234.8	110.0	47.4	142.2
Colorado	54.4	39.8	84.9	23.2	19.1	32.4	8.6	6.2	18.5
Connecticut	43.9	30.2	63.3	17.8	14.9	25.1	9.2	4.6	13.7
Delaware	13.9	9.3	18.7	5.6	5.1	8.2	3.3	1.1	3.3
District of Columbia	10.5	6.9	13.7	4.8	4.0	6.5	2.3	0.8	2.3
Florida	210.9	149.1	332.1	78.6	66.7	114.0	36.2	23.5	70.6
Georgia	116.5	77.3	169.2	44.4	36.2	61.6	24.5	12.2	36.5
Hawaii	15.2	12.4	25.3	7.1	6.6	10.9	1.9	1.7	5.0
Idaho	16.9	13.7	27.9	7.9	7.3	12.1	2.4	1.9	5.7
Illinois	157.0	106.4	232.4	63.3	49.2	83.7	27.4	16.7	50.0
Indiana	78.8	54.7	121.2	31.5	25.0	42.4	11.6	8.2	24.6
Iowa	36.7	26.6	57.0	16.0	12.8	21.5	4.8	3.9	11.6
Kansas	32.1	24.5	52.0	14.7	12.1	20.2	3.6	3.6	10.8
Kentucky	57.2	38.4	87.1	23.1	17.2	29.0	7.0	5.5	16.4
Louisiana	53.5	38.2	84.1	22.8	18.1	30.4	6.8	5.6	16.7
Maine	18.5	13.0	27.5	7.8	6.7	11.0	3.2	1.7	5.2
Maryland	63.3	46.8	99.8	24.6	22.5	38.2	12.2	7.3	21.9
Massachusetts	90.0	53.3	114.5	31.7	25.2	42.8	25.1	8.4	25.1
Michigan	121.2	85.5	188.8	49.9	39.2	66.7	16.8	13.1	39.4
Minnesota	58.4	43.4	92.2	24.7	20.8	35.2	9.1	6.7	20.2
Mississippi	39.2	26.7	59.4	15.8	12.7	21.3	6.2	3.8	11.4
Missouri	73.2	50.5	111.4	28.9	23.2	39.3	11.6	7.6	22.8
Montana	13.9	9.6	19.9	6.3	5.3	8.7	2.5	1.2	3.7
Nebraska	21.5	16.3	34.0	9.3	8.4	14.0	3.5	2.3	6.9
Nevada	32.5	22.6	48.7	13.5	11.0	18.5	5.4	3.2	9.7
New Hampshire	19.2	12.8	26.1	7.1	6.7	11.1	5.1	1.7	5.1
New Jersey	119.8	72.1	154.3	41.5	34.2	58.0	34.0	11.3	34.0
New Mexico	23.4	17.9	38.2	10.9	9.0	15.1	2.6	2.5	7.6
New York	254.3	155.1	339.4	89.9	71.3	121.9	66.1	25.1	75.3
North Carolina	106.8	74.3	165.1	42.9	33.8	57.6	16.2	11.5	34.5
North Dakota	9.3	7.2	14.5	4.7	4.2	6.8	1.2	0.8	2.5
Ohio	145.0	96.7	213.6	58.7	43.9	74.6	23.2	14.9	44.8
Oklahoma	45.0	32.2	71.7	19.3	15.0	25.3	4.8	4.7	14.0
Oregon	43.0	31.5	67.5	17.8	15.1	25.5	7.0	4.8	14.4
Pennsylvania	155.5	103.8	228.0	55.9	46.7	79.7	32.0	16.2	48.5
Rhode Island	15.2	10.8	22.5	6.7	5.8	9.6	2.7	1.4	4.2
South Carolina	62.2	37.7	83.1	20.5	17.7	29.8	16.9	5.6	16.9
South Dakota	11.3	8.5	17.0	5.5	4.8	7.7	1.5	1.0	3.0
Tennessee	71.7	51.8	115.0	28.2	23.7	40.2	10.6	7.9	23.6
Texas	266.3	189.4	411.2	114.1	90.2	153.4	43.1	30.6	91.7
Utah	23.6	21.1	42.0	11.6	11.6	19.4	3.7	3.3	9.9
Vermont	10.4	7.2	14.2	4.6	4.2	6.8	2.3	0.8	2.4
Virginia	103.2	63.5	137.0	33.4	29.6	50.3	29.8	9.9	29.8
Washington	67.3	52.5	111.8	28.9	25.0	42.5	9.2	8.3	24.9
West Virginia	27.8	17.6	38.7	10.4	8.4	14.0	5.7	2.4	7.1
Wisconsin	64.3	47.5	103.1	27.6	22.3	37.7	8.0	7.2	21.7
Wyoming	9.0	6.5	12.7	4.4	3.8	6.1	1.5	0.7	2.0

CDC Recommended Annual Total Funding Levels for State Programs, 2007

Cessation Interventions			Surveillance and Evaluation			Administration and Management			
Recommended (millions)	Lower (millions)	Upper (millions)	Recommended (millions)	Lower (millions)	Upper (millions)	Recommended (millions)	Lower (millions)	Upper (millions)	2006 Population Estimate (millions)
1,046.2	611.2	1,569.3	**321.4**	219.4	476.3	**161.0**	109.9	238.2	299.403
18.3	10.3	28.0	**4.9**	3.5	7.8	**2.5**	1.8	3.9	4.599
2.6	1.5	4.1	**0.9**	0.7	1.4	**0.5**	0.3	0.7	0.670
20.1	11.8	30.4	**5.9**	4.5	9.6	**3.0**	2.2	4.8	6.166
11.3	6.4	17.3	**3.2**	2.2	4.9	**1.6**	1.1	2.4	2.811
103.7	63.7	153.8	**38.4**	24.9	53.1	**19.2**	12.4	26.5	36.458
15.5	9.3	22.9	**4.7**	3.5	7.4	**2.4**	1.7	3.7	4.753
11.2	6.8	16.2	**3.8**	2.6	5.5	**1.9**	1.3	2.8	3.505
3.2	1.9	4.8	**1.2**	0.8	1.6	**0.6**	0.4	0.8	0.853
2.0	1.2	3.1	**0.9**	0.6	1.2	**0.5**	0.3	0.6	0.582
68.6	39.4	104.2	**18.3**	13.0	28.9	**9.2**	6.5	14.4	18.090
32.4	18.8	49.0	**10.1**	6.7	14.7	**5.1**	3.4	7.4	9.364
4.2	2.5	6.1	**1.3**	1.1	2.2	**0.7**	0.5	1.1	1.285
4.4	2.7	6.5	**1.5**	1.2	2.4	**0.7**	0.6	1.2	1.466
45.8	26.6	68.4	**13.7**	9.3	20.2	**6.8**	4.6	10.1	12.832
25.4	14.3	38.4	**6.9**	4.8	10.5	**3.4**	2.4	5.3	6.314
11.1	6.4	16.4	**3.2**	2.3	5.0	**1.6**	1.2	2.5	2.982
9.6	5.6	14.2	**2.8**	2.1	4.5	**1.4**	1.1	2.3	2.764
19.6	10.7	30.3	**5.0**	3.3	7.6	**2.5**	1.7	3.8	4.206
16.9	9.5	26.0	**4.7**	3.3	7.3	**2.3**	1.7	3.7	4.288
5.1	2.9	7.7	**1.6**	1.1	2.4	**0.8**	0.6	1.2	1.322
18.2	10.9	26.7	**5.5**	4.1	8.7	**2.8**	2.0	4.3	5.616
21.5	12.8	31.6	**7.8**	4.6	10.0	**3.9**	2.3	5.0	6.437
38.7	22.1	58.1	**10.5**	7.4	16.4	**5.3**	3.7	8.2	10.096
17.0	10.2	24.8	**5.1**	3.8	8.0	**2.5**	1.9	4.0	5.167
12.1	6.7	18.9	**3.4**	2.3	5.2	**1.7**	1.2	2.6	2.911
23.1	13.1	34.8	**6.4**	4.4	9.7	**3.2**	2.2	4.8	5.843
3.3	1.9	4.9	**1.2**	0.8	1.7	**0.6**	0.4	0.9	0.945
5.9	3.5	8.6	**1.9**	1.4	3.0	**0.9**	0.7	1.5	1.768
9.4	5.4	14.2	**2.8**	2.0	4.2	**1.4**	1.0	2.1	2.496
4.5	2.7	6.5	**1.7**	1.1	2.3	**0.8**	0.6	1.1	1.315
28.7	17.2	42.2	**10.4**	6.3	13.4	**5.2**	3.1	6.7	8.725
6.9	4.0	10.5	**2.0**	1.6	3.3	**1.0**	0.8	1.7	1.955
65.1	38.5	97.9	**22.1**	13.5	29.5	**11.1**	6.7	14.8	19.306
33.8	19.3	51.4	**9.3**	6.5	14.4	**4.6**	3.2	7.2	8.857
2.2	1.3	3.3	**0.8**	0.6	1.3	**0.4**	0.3	0.6	0.636
44.2	25.3	66.3	**12.6**	8.4	18.6	**6.3**	4.2	9.3	11.478
15.0	8.3	23.1	**3.9**	2.8	6.2	**2.0**	1.4	3.1	3.579
12.6	7.5	18.8	**3.7**	2.7	5.9	**1.9**	1.4	2.9	3.701
47.3	27.4	70.1	**13.5**	9.0	19.8	**6.8**	4.5	9.9	12.441
3.8	2.2	5.7	**1.3**	0.9	2.0	**0.7**	0.5	1.0	1.068
16.7	9.5	25.6	**5.4**	3.3	7.2	**2.7**	1.6	3.6	4.321
2.8	1.6	4.1	**1.0**	0.7	1.5	**0.5**	0.4	0.7	0.782
23.6	13.4	36.2	**6.2**	4.5	10.0	**3.1**	2.3	5.0	6.039
74.3	43.9	112.4	**23.2**	16.5	35.8	**11.6**	8.2	17.9	23.508
5.2	3.5	7.2	**2.1**	1.8	3.7	**1.0**	0.9	1.8	2.550
2.1	1.3	3.2	**0.9**	0.6	1.2	**0.5**	0.3	0.6	0.624
26.5	15.7	39.0	**9.0**	5.5	11.9	**4.5**	2.8	6.0	7.643
20.4	12.3	29.8	**5.9**	4.6	9.7	**2.9**	2.3	4.9	6.396
8.1	4.5	12.5	**2.4**	1.5	3.4	**1.2**	0.8	1.7	1.818
20.3	11.8	30.2	**5.6**	4.1	9.0	**2.8**	2.1	4.5	5.557
1.9	1.1	2.9	**0.8**	0.6	1.1	**0.4**	0.3	0.6	0.515

Section C

CDC Recommended Annual Investment $56.7 million

Deaths in Alabama Caused by Smoking

Annual average smoking-attributable deaths	7,400
Youth ages 0-17 projected to die from smoking	174,000

Annual Costs Incurred in Alabama from Smoking

Total medical	$1,499 million
Medicaid medical	$238 million
Lost productivity from premature death	$2,051 million

State Revenue from Tobacco Excise Taxes and Settlement

FY 2006 tobacco tax revenue	$156.2 million
FY 2006 tobacco settlement payment	$94.3 million

Total state revenue from tobacco excise taxes and settlement $250.5 million

Percent tobacco revenue to fund at CDC recommended level   23%

	Per Capita Recommendation
I. State and Community Interventions Multiple societal resources working together have the greatest long-term population impact.	**$5.04**
II. Health Communication Interventions Media interventions prevent tobacco use initiation, promote cessation, and shape social norms.	**$1.69**
III. Cessation Interventions Tobacco use treatment is highly cost-effective.	**$3.97**
IV. Surveillance and Evaluation Publicly financed programs should be accountable and demonstrate effectiveness.	**$1.07**
V. Administration and Management Complex, integrated programs require experienced staff to provide fiscal management, accountability, and coordination.	**$0.54**
Total	**$12.31**

Note: *A justification for each program element and the rationale for the budget estimates are provided in Section A. The funding estimates presented are based on adjustments for changes in population and inflation since the 1999 publication. The recommended levels of investment (per capita and total) are presented in 2007 dollars using 2006 population estimates. These should be updated annually according to the U.S. Department of Labor Consumer Price Index and U.S. Census Bureau. The actual funding required for implementing programs will vary depending on state characteristics such as tobacco use prevalence, socio-demographic factors, and other factors. See Appendix E for data sources on deaths, costs, revenue and state-specific factors.*

Office on Smoking and Health • Centers for Disease Control and Prevention
www.cdc.gov/tobacco • tobaccoinfo@cdc.gov • 1 (800) CDC INFO or 1 (800) 232-4636

CDC Recommended Annual Investment $10.7 million

Deaths in Alaska Caused by Smoking

Annual average smoking-attributable deaths	500
Youth ages 0-17 projected to die from smoking	18,000

Annual Costs Incurred in Alaska from Smoking

Total medical	$169 million
Medicaid medical	$77 million
Lost productivity from premature death	$157 million

State Revenue from Tobacco Excise Taxes and Settlement

FY 2006 tobacco tax revenue	$65.2 million
FY 2006 tobacco settlement payment	$19.9 million
Total state revenue from tobacco excise taxes and settlement	$85.1 million

Percent tobacco revenue to fund at CDC recommended level   13%

	Per Capita Recommendation
I. State and Community Interventions Multiple societal resources working together have the greatest long-term population impact.	**$7.93**
II. Health Communication Interventions Media interventions prevent tobacco use initiation, promote cessation, and shape social norms.	**$2.13**
III. Cessation Interventions Tobacco use treatment is highly cost-effective.	**$3.95**
IV. Surveillance and Evaluation Publicly financed programs should be accountable and demonstrate effectiveness.	**$1.40**
V. Administration and Management Complex, integrated programs require experienced staff to provide fiscal management, accountability, and coordination.	**$0.70**
Total	**$16.11**

Note: A justification for each program element and the rationale for the budget estimates are provided in Section A. The funding estimates presented are based on adjustments for changes in population and inflation since the 1999 publication. The recommended levels of investment (per capita and total) are presented in 2007 dollars using 2006 population estimates. These should be updated annually according to the U.S. Department of Labor Consumer Price Index and U.S. Census Bureau. The actual funding required for implementing programs will vary depending on state characteristics such as tobacco use prevalence, socio-demographic factors, and other factors. See Appendix E for data sources on deaths, costs, revenue and state-specific factors.

Office on Smoking and Health • Centers for Disease Control and Prevention
www.cdc.gov/tobacco • tobaccoinfo@cdc.gov • 1 (800) CDC INFO or 1 (800) 232-4636

Arizona

CDC Recommended Annual Investment $68.1 million

Deaths in Arizona Caused by Smoking

Annual average smoking-attributable deaths	6,300
Youth ages 0-17 projected to die from smoking	105,000

Annual Costs Incurred in Arizona from Smoking

Total medical	$1,287 million
Medicaid medical	$316 million
Lost productivity from premature death	$1,492 million

State Revenue from Tobacco Excise Taxes and Settlement

FY 2006 tobacco tax revenue	$302.5 million
FY 2006 tobacco settlement payment	$86.0 million
Total state revenue from tobacco excise taxes and settlement	$388.5 million

Percent tobacco revenue to fund at CDC recommended level   18%

	Per Capita Recommendation
I. State and Community Interventions Multiple societal resources working together have the greatest long-term population impact.	$4.70
II. Health Communication Interventions Media interventions prevent tobacco use initiation, promote cessation, and shape social norms.	$1.64
III. Cessation Interventions Tobacco use treatment is highly cost-effective.	$3.25
IV. Surveillance and Evaluation Publicly financed programs should be accountable and demonstrate effectiveness.	$0.96
V. Administration and Management Complex, integrated programs require experienced staff to provide fiscal management, accountability, and coordination.	$0.48
Total	**$11.03**

Note: A justification for each program element and the rationale for the budget estimates are provided in Section A. The funding estimates presented are based on adjustments for changes in population and inflation since the 1999 publication. The recommended levels of investment (per capita and total) are presented in 2007 dollars using 2006 population estimates. These should be updated annually according to the U.S. Department of Labor Consumer Price Index and U.S. Census Bureau. The actual funding required for implementing programs will vary depending on state characteristics such as tobacco use prevalence, socio-demographic factors, and other factors. See Appendix E for data sources on deaths, costs, revenue and state-specific factors.

Office on Smoking and Health • Centers for Disease Control and Prevention
www.cdc.gov/tobacco • tobaccoinfo@cdc.gov • 1 (800) CDC INFO or 1 (800) 232-4636

CDC Recommended Annual Investment $36.4 million

Deaths in Arkansas Caused by Smoking

Annual average smoking-attributable deaths	4,900
Youth ages 0-17 projected to die from smoking	64,000

Annual Costs Incurred in Arkansas from Smoking

Total medical	$812 million
Medicaid medical	$242 million
Lost productivity from premature death	$1,306 million

State Revenue from Tobacco Excise Taxes and Settlement

FY 2006 tobacco tax revenue	$148.8 million
FY 2006 tobacco settlement payment	$48.3 million
Total state revenue from tobacco excise taxes and settlement	$197.1 million

Percent tobacco revenue to fund at CDC recommended level   18%

	Per Capita Recommendation
I. State and Community Interventions Multiple societal resources working together have the greatest long-term population impact.	**$5.43**
II. Health Communication Interventions Media interventions prevent tobacco use initiation, promote cessation, and shape social norms.	**$1.78**
III. Cessation Interventions Tobacco use treatment is highly cost-effective.	**$4.02**
IV. Surveillance and Evaluation Publicly financed programs should be accountable and demonstrate effectiveness.	**$1.12**
V. Administration and Management Complex, integrated programs require experienced staff to provide fiscal management, accountability, and coordination.	**$0.56**
Total	**$12.91**

Note: A justification for each program element and the rationale for the budget estimates are provided in Section A. The funding estimates presented are based on adjustments for changes in population and inflation since the 1999 publication. The recommended levels of investment (per capita and total) are presented in 2007 dollars using 2006 population estimates. These should be updated annually according to the U.S. Department of Labor Consumer Price Index and U.S. Census Bureau. The actual funding required for implementing programs will vary depending on state characteristics such as tobacco use prevalence, socio-demographic factors, and other factors. See Appendix E for data sources on deaths, costs, revenue and state-specific factors.

Office on Smoking and Health • Centers for Disease Control and Prevention
www.cdc.gov/tobacco • tobaccoinfo@cdc.gov • 1 (800) CDC INFO or 1 (800) 232-4636

CDC Recommended Annual Investment $441.9 million

Deaths in California Caused by Smoking

Annual average smoking-attributable deaths	37,800
Youth ages 0-17 projected to die from smoking	596,000

Annual Costs Incurred in California from Smoking

Total medical	$9,142 million
Medicaid medical	$2,959 million
Lost productivity from premature death	$8,585 million

State Revenue from Tobacco Excise Taxes and Settlement

FY 2006 tobacco tax revenue	$1,084.3 million
FY 2006 tobacco settlement payment	$744.5 million
Total state revenue from tobacco excise taxes and settlement	$1,828.8 million

Percent tobacco revenue to fund at CDC recommended level   24%

	Per Capita Recommendation
I. State and Community Interventions Multiple societal resources working together have the greatest long-term population impact.	**$4.68**
II. Health Communication Interventions Media interventions prevent tobacco use initiation, promote cessation, and shape social norms.	**$3.02**
III. Cessation Interventions Tobacco use treatment is highly cost-effective.	**$2.84**
IV. Surveillance and Evaluation Publicly financed programs should be accountable and demonstrate effectiveness.	**$1.05**
V. Administration and Management Complex, integrated programs require experienced staff to provide fiscal management, accountability, and coordination.	**$0.53**
Total	**$12.12**

Note: A justification for each program element and the rationale for the budget estimates are provided in Section A. The funding estimates presented are based on adjustments for changes in population and inflation since the 1999 publication. The recommended levels of investment (per capita and total) are presented in 2007 dollars using 2006 population estimates. These should be updated annually according to the U.S. Department of Labor Consumer Price Index and U.S. Census Bureau. The actual funding required for implementing programs will vary depending on state characteristics such as tobacco use prevalence, socio-demographic factors, and other factors. See Appendix E for data sources on deaths, costs, revenue and state-specific factors.

Office on Smoking and Health • Centers for Disease Control and Prevention
www.cdc.gov/tobacco • tobaccoinfo@cdc.gov • 1 (800) CDC INFO or 1 (800) 232-4636

CDC Recommended Annual Investment $54.4 million

Deaths in Colorado Caused by Smoking

Annual average smoking-attributable deaths	4,300
Youth ages 0-17 projected to die from smoking	92,000

Annual Costs Incurred in Colorado from Smoking

Total medical	$1,314 million
Medicaid medical	$319 million
Lost productivity from premature death	$992 million

State Revenue from Tobacco Excise Taxes and Settlement

FY 2006 tobacco tax revenue	$229.2 million
FY 2006 tobacco settlement payment	$80.0 million
Total state revenue from tobacco excise taxes and settlement	$309.2 million

Percent tobacco revenue to fund at CDC recommended level   18%

	Per Capita Recommendation
I. State and Community Interventions Multiple societal resources working together have the greatest long-term population impact.	**$4.89**
II. Health Communication Interventions Media interventions prevent tobacco use initiation, promote cessation, and shape social norms.	**$1.81**
III. Cessation Interventions Tobacco use treatment is highly cost-effective.	**$3.26**
IV. Surveillance and Evaluation Publicly financed programs should be accountable and demonstrate effectiveness.	**$1.00**
V. Administration and Management Complex, integrated programs require experienced staff to provide fiscal management, accountability, and coordination.	**$0.50**
Total	**$11.46**

Note: A justification for each program element and the rationale for the budget estimates are provided in Section A. The funding estimates presented are based on adjustments for changes in population and inflation since the 1999 publication. The recommended levels of investment (per capita and total) are presented in 2007 dollars using 2006 population estimates. These should be updated annually according to the U.S. Department of Labor Consumer Price Index and U.S. Census Bureau. The actual funding required for implementing programs will vary depending on state characteristics such as tobacco use prevalence, socio-demographic factors, and other factors. See Appendix E for data sources on deaths, costs, revenue and state-specific factors.

Office on Smoking and Health • Centers for Disease Control and Prevention
www.cdc.gov/tobacco • tobaccoinfo@cdc.gov • 1 (800) CDC INFO or 1 (800) 232-4636

CDC Recommended Annual Investment $43.9 million

Deaths in Connecticut Caused by Smoking

Annual average smoking-attributable deaths	4,900
Youth ages 0-17 projected to die from smoking	76,000

Annual Costs Incurred in Connecticut from Smoking

Total medical	$1,631 million
Medicaid medical	$430 million
Lost productivity from premature death	$1,017 million

State Revenue from Tobacco Excise Taxes and Settlement

FY 2006 tobacco tax revenue	$272.2 million
FY 2006 tobacco settlement payment	$108.3 million

Total state revenue from tobacco excise taxes and settlement $380.5 million

Percent tobacco revenue to fund at CDC recommended level   12%

	Per Capita Recommendation
I. State and Community Interventions Multiple societal resources working together have the greatest long-term population impact.	**$5.09**
II. Health Communication Interventions Media interventions prevent tobacco use initiation, promote cessation, and shape social norms.	**$2.63**
III. Cessation Interventions Tobacco use treatment is highly cost-effective.	**$3.18**
IV. Surveillance and Evaluation Publicly financed programs should be accountable and demonstrate effectiveness.	**$1.09**
V. Administration and Management Complex, integrated programs require experienced staff to provide fiscal management, accountability, and coordination.	**$0.55**
Total	**$12.54**

Note: A justification for each program element and the rationale for the budget estimates are provided in Section A. The funding estimates presented are based on adjustments for changes in population and inflation since the 1999 publication. The recommended levels of investment (per capita and total) are presented in 2007 dollars using 2006 population estimates. These should be updated annually according to the U.S. Department of Labor Consumer Price Index and U.S. Census Bureau. The actual funding required for implementing programs will vary depending on state characteristics such as tobacco use prevalence, socio-demographic factors, and other factors. See Appendix E for data sources on deaths, costs, revenue and state-specific factors.

Office on Smoking and Health • Centers for Disease Control and Prevention
www.cdc.gov/tobacco • tobaccoinfo@cdc.gov • 1 (800) CDC INFO or 1 (800) 232-4636

CDC Recommended Annual Investment $13.9 million

Deaths in Delaware Caused by Smoking

Annual average smoking-attributable deaths	1,200
Youth ages 0-17 projected to die from smoking	18,000

Annual Costs Incurred in Delaware from Smoking

Total medical	$284 million
Medicaid medical	$79 million
Lost productivity from premature death	$304 million

State Revenue from Tobacco Excise Taxes and Settlement

FY 2006 tobacco tax revenue	$86.1 million
FY 2006 tobacco settlement payment	$23.1 million
Total state revenue from tobacco excise taxes and settlement	$109.2 million

Percent tobacco revenue to fund at CDC recommended level   13%

	Per Capita Recommendation
I. State and Community Interventions Multiple societal resources working together have the greatest long-term population impact.	**$6.52**
II. Health Communication Interventions Media interventions prevent tobacco use initiation, promote cessation, and shape social norms.	**$3.90**
III. Cessation Interventions Tobacco use treatment is highly cost-effective.	**$3.77**
IV. Surveillance and Evaluation Publicly financed programs should be accountable and demonstrate effectiveness.	**$1.42**
V. Administration and Management Complex, integrated programs require experienced staff to provide fiscal management, accountability, and coordination.	**$0.71**
Total	**$16.32**

Note: *A justification for each program element and the rationale for the budget estimates are provided in Section A. The funding estimates presented are based on adjustments for changes in population and inflation since the 1999 publication. The recommended levels of investment (per capita and total) are presented in 2007 dollars using 2006 population estimates. These should be updated annually according to the U.S. Department of Labor Consumer Price Index and U.S. Census Bureau. The actual funding required for implementing programs will vary depending on state characteristics such as tobacco use prevalence, socio-demographic factors, and other factors. See Appendix E for data sources on deaths, costs, revenue and state-specific factors.*

Office on Smoking and Health • Centers for Disease Control and Prevention
www.cdc.gov/tobacco • tobaccoinfo@cdc.gov • 1 (800) CDC INFO or 1 (800) 232-4636

District of Columbia

CDC Recommended Annual Investment $10.5 million

Deaths in District of Columbia Caused by Smoking

Annual average smoking-attributable deaths	700
Youth ages 0-17 projected to die from smoking	8,000

Annual Costs Incurred in District of Columbia from Smoking

Total medical	$243 million
Medicaid medical	$78 million
Lost productivity from premature death	$233 million

State Revenue from Tobacco Excise Taxes and Settlement

FY 2006 tobacco tax revenue	$22.8 million
FY 2006 tobacco settlement payment	$35.4 million
Total state revenue from tobacco excise taxes and settlement	$58.2 million

Percent tobacco revenue to fund at CDC recommended level   18%

	Per Capita Recommendation
I. State and Community Interventions Multiple societal resources working together have the greatest long-term population impact.	$8.27
II. Health Communication Interventions Media interventions prevent tobacco use initiation, promote cessation, and shape social norms.	$3.90
III. Cessation Interventions Tobacco use treatment is highly cost-effective.	$3.50
IV. Surveillance and Evaluation Publicly financed programs should be accountable and demonstrate effectiveness.	$1.57
V. Administration and Management Complex, integrated programs require experienced staff to provide fiscal management, accountability, and coordination.	$0.78
Total	**$18.02**

Note: A justification for each program element and the rationale for the budget estimates are provided in Section A. The funding estimates presented are based on adjustments for changes in population and inflation since the 1999 publication. The recommended levels of investment (per capita and total) are presented in 2007 dollars using 2006 population estimates. These should be updated annually according to the U.S. Department of Labor Consumer Price Index and U.S. Census Bureau. The actual funding required for implementing programs will vary depending on state characteristics such as tobacco use prevalence, socio-demographic factors, and other factors. See Appendix E for data sources on deaths, costs, revenue and state-specific factors.

Office on Smoking and Health • Centers for Disease Control and Prevention
www.cdc.gov/tobacco • tobaccoinfo@cdc.gov • 1 (800) CDC INFO or 1 (800) 232-4636

CDC Recommended Annual Investment $210.9 million

Deaths in Florida Caused by Smoking

Annual average smoking-attributable deaths	28,700
Youth ages 0-17 projected to die from smoking	369,000

Annual Costs Incurred in Florida from Smoking

Total medical	$6,320 million
Medicaid medical	$1,250 million
Lost productivity from premature death	$6,479 million

State Revenue from Tobacco Excise Taxes and Settlement

FY 2006 tobacco tax revenue	$451.8 million
FY 2006 tobacco settlement payment	$380.2 million

Total state revenue from tobacco excise taxes and settlement $832.0 million

Percent tobacco revenue to fund at CDC recommended level   25%

	Per Capita Recommendation
I. State and Community Interventions Multiple societal resources working together have the greatest long-term population impact.	**$4.35**
II. Health Communication Interventions Media interventions prevent tobacco use initiation, promote cessation, and shape social norms.	**$2.00**
III. Cessation Interventions Tobacco use treatment is highly cost-effective.	**$3.79**
IV. Surveillance and Evaluation Publicly financed programs should be accountable and demonstrate effectiveness.	**$1.01**
V. Administration and Management Complex, integrated programs require experienced staff to provide fiscal management, accountability, and coordination.	**$0.51**
Total	**$11.66**

Note: A justification for each program element and the rationale for the budget estimates are provided in Section A. The funding estimates presented are based on adjustments for changes in population and inflation since the 1999 publication. The recommended levels of investment (per capita and total) are presented in 2007 dollars using 2006 population estimates. These should be updated annually according to the U.S. Department of Labor Consumer Price Index and U.S. Census Bureau. The actual funding required for implementing programs will vary depending on state characteristics such as tobacco use prevalence, socio-demographic factors, and other factors. See Appendix E for data sources on deaths, costs, revenue and state-specific factors.

Office on Smoking and Health • Centers for Disease Control and Prevention
www.cdc.gov/tobacco • tobaccoinfo@cdc.gov • 1 (800) CDC INFO or 1 (800) 232-4636

CDC Recommended Annual Investment $116.5 million

Deaths in Georgia Caused by Smoking

Annual average smoking-attributable deaths	10,300
Youth ages 0-17 projected to die from smoking	184,000

Annual Costs Incurred in Georgia from Smoking

Total medical	$2,252 million
Medicaid medical	$537 million
Lost productivity from premature death	$3,082 million

State Revenue from Tobacco Excise Taxes and Settlement

FY 2006 tobacco tax revenue	$248.0 million
FY 2006 tobacco settlement payment	$143.2 million

Total state revenue from tobacco excise taxes and settlement $391.2 million

Percent tobacco revenue to fund at CDC recommended level   30%

	Per Capita Recommendation
I. State and Community Interventions Multiple societal resources working together have the greatest long-term population impact.	$4.74
II. Health Communication Interventions Media interventions prevent tobacco use initiation, promote cessation, and shape social norms.	$2.62
III. Cessation Interventions Tobacco use treatment is highly cost-effective.	$3.46
IV. Surveillance and Evaluation Publicly financed programs should be accountable and demonstrate effectiveness.	$1.08
V. Administration and Management Complex, integrated programs require experienced staff to provide fiscal management, accountability, and coordination.	$0.54
Total	**$12.44**

Note: A justification for each program element and the rationale for the budget estimates are provided in Section A. The funding estimates presented are based on adjustments for changes in population and inflation since the 1999 publication. The recommended levels of investment (per capita and total) are presented in 2007 dollars using 2006 population estimates. These should be updated annually according to the U.S. Department of Labor Consumer Price Index and U.S. Census Bureau. The actual funding required for implementing programs will vary depending on state characteristics such as tobacco use prevalence, socio-demographic factors, and other factors. See Appendix E for data sources on deaths, costs, revenue and state-specific factors.

Office on Smoking and Health • Centers for Disease Control and Prevention
www.cdc.gov/tobacco • tobaccoinfo@cdc.gov • 1 (800) CDC INFO or 1 (800) 232-4636

CDC Recommended Annual Investment $15.2 million

Deaths in Hawaii Caused by Smoking

Annual average smoking-attributable deaths	1,200
Youth ages 0-17 projected to die from smoking	NA

Annual Costs Incurred in Hawaii from Smoking

Total medical	$336 million
Medicaid medical	$117 million
Lost productivity from premature death	$308 million

State Revenue from Tobacco Excise Taxes and Settlement

FY 2006 tobacco tax revenue	$88.3 million
FY 2006 tobacco settlement payment	$35.1 million
Total state revenue from tobacco excise taxes and settlement	$123.4 million

Percent tobacco revenue to fund at CDC recommended level   12%

		Per Capita Recommendation
I.	**State and Community Interventions** Multiple societal resources working together have the greatest long-term population impact.	**$5.55**
II.	**Health Communication Interventions** Media interventions prevent tobacco use initiation, promote cessation, and shape social norms.	**$1.46**
III.	**Cessation Interventions** Tobacco use treatment is highly cost-effective.	**$3.25**
IV.	**Surveillance and Evaluation** Publicly financed programs should be accountable and demonstrate effectiveness.	**$1.03**
V.	**Administration and Management** Complex, integrated programs require experienced staff to provide fiscal management, accountability, and coordination.	**$0.51**
	Total	**$11.80**

Note: A justification for each program element and the rationale for the budget estimates are provided in Section A. The funding estimates presented are based on adjustments for changes in population and inflation since the 1999 publication. The recommended levels of investment (per capita and total) are presented in 2007 dollars using 2006 population estimates. These should be updated annually according to the U.S. Department of Labor Consumer Price Index and U.S. Census Bureau. The actual funding required for implementing programs will vary depending on state characteristics such as tobacco use prevalence, socio-demographic factors, and other factors. See Appendix E for data sources on deaths, costs, revenue and state-specific factors.

Office on Smoking and Health • Centers for Disease Control and Prevention
www.cdc.gov/tobacco • tobaccoinfo@cdc.gov • 1 (800) CDC INFO or 1 (800) 232-4636

Idaho

CDC Recommended Annual Investment $16.9 million

Deaths in Idaho Caused by Smoking

Annual average smoking-attributable deaths	1,500
Youth ages 0-17 projected to die from smoking	24,000

Annual Costs Incurred in Idaho from Smoking

Total medical	$319 million
Medicaid medical	$83 million
Lost productivity from premature death	$333 million

State Revenue from Tobacco Excise Taxes and Settlement

FY 2006 tobacco tax revenue	$53.4 million
FY 2006 tobacco settlement payment	$21.2 million
Total state revenue from tobacco excise taxes and settlement	$74.6 million

Percent tobacco revenue to fund at CDC recommended level   23%

	Per Capita Recommendation
I. State and Community Interventions Multiple societal resources working together have the greatest long-term population impact.	$5.36
II. Health Communication Interventions Media interventions prevent tobacco use initiation, promote cessation, and shape social norms.	$1.61
III. Cessation Interventions Tobacco use treatment is highly cost-effective.	$3.03
IV. Surveillance and Evaluation Publicly financed programs should be accountable and demonstrate effectiveness.	$1.00
V. Administration and Management Complex, integrated programs require experienced staff to provide fiscal management, accountability, and coordination.	$0.50
Total	**$11.50**

Note: A justification for each program element and the rationale for the budget estimates are provided in Section A. The funding estimates presented are based on adjustments for changes in population and inflation since the 1999 publication. The recommended levels of investment (per capita and total) are presented in 2007 dollars using 2006 population estimates. These should be updated annually according to the U.S. Department of Labor Consumer Price Index and U.S. Census Bureau. The actual funding required for implementing programs will vary depending on state characteristics such as tobacco use prevalence, socio-demographic factors, and other factors. See Appendix E for data sources on deaths, costs, revenue and state-specific factors.

Office on Smoking and Health • Centers for Disease Control and Prevention
www.cdc.gov/tobacco • tobaccoinfo@cdc.gov • 1 (800) CDC INFO or 1 (800) 232-4636

CDC Recommended Annual Investment $157.0 million

Deaths in Illinois Caused by Smoking

Annual average smoking-attributable deaths	16,900
Youth ages 0-17 projected to die from smoking	317,000

Annual Costs Incurred in Illinois from Smoking

Total medical	$4,106 million
Medicaid medical	$1,570 million
Lost productivity from premature death	$4,292 million

State Revenue from Tobacco Excise Taxes and Settlement

FY 2006 tobacco tax revenue	$653.1 million
FY 2006 tobacco settlement payment	$271.5 million

Total state revenue from tobacco excise taxes and settlement $924.6 million

Percent tobacco revenue to fund at CDC recommended level   17%

	Per Capita Recommendation
I. State and Community Interventions Multiple societal resources working together have the greatest long-term population impact.	**$4.93**
II. Health Communication Interventions Media interventions prevent tobacco use initiation, promote cessation, and shape social norms.	**$2.14**
III. Cessation Interventions Tobacco use treatment is highly cost-effective.	**$3.57**
IV. Surveillance and Evaluation Publicly financed programs should be accountable and demonstrate effectiveness.	**$1.06**
V. Administration and Management Complex, integrated programs require experienced staff to provide fiscal management, accountability, and coordination.	**$0.53**
Total	**$12.23**

Note: A justification for each program element and the rationale for the budget estimates are provided in Section A. The funding estimates presented are based on adjustments for changes in population and inflation since the 1999 publication. The recommended levels of investment (per capita and total) are presented in 2007 dollars using 2006 population estimates. These should be updated annually according to the U.S. Department of Labor Consumer Price Index and U.S. Census Bureau. The actual funding required for implementing programs will vary depending on state characteristics such as tobacco use prevalence, socio-demographic factors, and other factors. See Appendix E for data sources on deaths, costs, revenue and state-specific factors.

Office on Smoking and Health • Centers for Disease Control and Prevention
www.cdc.gov/tobacco • tobaccoinfo@cdc.gov • 1 (800) CDC INFO or 1 (800) 232-4636

CDC Recommended Annual Investment $78.8 million

Deaths in Indiana Caused by Smoking

Annual average smoking-attributable deaths	9,800
Youth ages 0-17 projected to die from smoking	160,000

Annual Costs Incurred in Indiana from Smoking

Total medical	$2,084 million
Medicaid medical	$487 million
Lost productivity from premature death	$2,495 million

State Revenue from Tobacco Excise Taxes and Settlement

FY 2006 tobacco tax revenue	$356.1 million
FY 2006 tobacco settlement payment	$119.0 million

Total state revenue from tobacco excise taxes and settlement $475.1 million

Percent tobacco revenue to fund at CDC recommended level   17%

		Per Capita Recommendation
I.	**State and Community Interventions** Multiple societal resources working together have the greatest long-term population impact.	**$4.99**
II.	**Health Communication Interventions** Media interventions prevent tobacco use initiation, promote cessation, and shape social norms.	**$1.83**
III.	**Cessation Interventions** Tobacco use treatment is highly cost-effective.	**$4.02**
IV.	**Surveillance and Evaluation** Publicly financed programs should be accountable and demonstrate effectiveness.	**$1.08**
V.	**Administration and Management** Complex, integrated programs require experienced staff to provide fiscal management, accountability, and coordination.	**$0.54**
	Total	**$12.46**

Note: A justification for each program element and the rationale for the budget estimates are provided in Section A. The funding estimates presented are based on adjustments for changes in population and inflation since the 1999 publication. The recommended levels of investment (per capita and total) are presented in 2007 dollars using 2006 population estimates. These should be updated annually according to the U.S. Department of Labor Consumer Price Index and U.S. Census Bureau. The actual funding required for implementing programs will vary depending on state characteristics such as tobacco use prevalence, socio-demographic factors, and other factors. See Appendix E for data sources on deaths, costs, revenue and state-specific factors.

Office on Smoking and Health • Centers for Disease Control and Prevention
www.cdc.gov/tobacco • tobaccoinfo@cdc.gov • 1 (800) CDC INFO or 1 (800) 232-4636

CDC Recommended Annual Investment $36.7 million

Deaths in Iowa Caused by Smoking

Annual average smoking-attributable deaths	4,500
Youth ages 0-17 projected to die from smoking	66,000

Annual Costs Incurred in Iowa from Smoking

Total medical	$1,017 million
Medicaid medical	$301 million
Lost productivity from premature death	$963 million

State Revenue from Tobacco Excise Taxes and Settlement

FY 2006 tobacco tax revenue	$98.7 million
FY 2006 tobacco settlement payment	$50.7 million
Total state revenue from tobacco excise taxes and settlement	$149.4 million

Percent tobacco revenue to fund at CDC recommended level   25%

	Per Capita Recommendation
I. State and Community Interventions Multiple societal resources working together have the greatest long-term population impact.	$5.37
II. Health Communication Interventions Media interventions prevent tobacco use initiation, promote cessation, and shape social norms.	$1.60
III. Cessation Interventions Tobacco use treatment is highly cost-effective.	$3.72
IV. Surveillance and Evaluation Publicly financed programs should be accountable and demonstrate effectiveness.	$1.07
V. Administration and Management Complex, integrated programs require experienced staff to provide fiscal management, accountability, and coordination.	$0.53
Total	**$12.29**

Note: A justification for each program element and the rationale for the budget estimates are provided in Section A. The funding estimates presented are based on adjustments for changes in population and inflation since the 1999 publication. The recommended levels of investment (per capita and total) are presented in 2007 dollars using 2006 population estimates. These should be updated annually according to the U.S. Department of Labor Consumer Price Index and U.S. Census Bureau. The actual funding required for implementing programs will vary depending on state characteristics such as tobacco use prevalence, socio-demographic factors, and other factors. See Appendix E for data sources on deaths, costs, revenue and state-specific factors.

Office on Smoking and Health • Centers for Disease Control and Prevention
www.cdc.gov/tobacco • tobaccoinfo@cdc.gov • 1 (800) CDC INFO or 1 (800) 232-4636

CDC Recommended Annual Investment $32.1 million

Deaths in Kansas Caused by Smoking

Annual average smoking-attributable deaths	3,900
Youth ages 0-17 projected to die from smoking	54,000

Annual Costs Incurred in Kansas from Smoking

Total medical	$927 million
Medicaid medical	$196 million
Lost productivity from premature death	$863 million

State Revenue from Tobacco Excise Taxes and Settlement

FY 2006 tobacco tax revenue	$124.0 million
FY 2006 tobacco settlement payment	$48.6 million
Total state revenue from tobacco excise taxes and settlement	$172.6 million

Percent tobacco revenue to fund at CDC recommended level   19%

	Per Capita Recommendation
I. State and Community Interventions Multiple societal resources working together have the greatest long-term population impact.	$5.31
II. Health Communication Interventions Media interventions prevent tobacco use initiation, promote cessation, and shape social norms.	$1.30
III. Cessation Interventions Tobacco use treatment is highly cost-effective.	$3.48
IV. Surveillance and Evaluation Publicly financed programs should be accountable and demonstrate effectiveness.	$1.01
V. Administration and Management Complex, integrated programs require experienced staff to provide fiscal management, accountability, and coordination.	$0.50
Total	**$11.60**

Note: A justification for each program element and the rationale for the budget estimates are provided in Section A. The funding estimates presented are based on adjustments for changes in population and inflation since the 1999 publication. The recommended levels of investment (per capita and total) are presented in 2007 dollars using 2006 population estimates. These should be updated annually according to the U.S. Department of Labor Consumer Price Index and U.S. Census Bureau. The actual funding required for implementing programs will vary depending on state characteristics such as tobacco use prevalence, socio-demographic factors, and other factors. See Appendix E for data sources on deaths, costs, revenue and state-specific factors.

Office on Smoking and Health • Centers for Disease Control and Prevention
www.cdc.gov/tobacco • tobaccoinfo@cdc.gov • 1 (800) CDC INFO or 1 (800) 232-4636

CDC Recommended Annual Investment $57.2 million

Deaths in Kentucky Caused by Smoking

Annual average smoking-attributable deaths	7,700
Youth ages 0-17 projected to die from smoking	107,000

Annual Costs Incurred in Kentucky from Smoking

Total medical	$1,500 million
Medicaid medical	$487 million
Lost productivity from premature death	$2,138 million

State Revenue from Tobacco Excise Taxes and Settlement

FY 2006 tobacco tax revenue	$165.2 million
FY 2006 tobacco settlement payment	$102.7 million

Total state revenue from tobacco excise taxes and settlement $267.9 million

Percent tobacco revenue to fund at CDC recommended level 21%

	Per Capita Recommendation
I. State and Community Interventions Multiple societal resources working together have the greatest long-term population impact.	**$5.50**
II. Health Communication Interventions Media interventions prevent tobacco use initiation, promote cessation, and shape social norms.	**$1.65**
III. Cessation Interventions Tobacco use treatment is highly cost-effective.	**$4.67**
IV. Surveillance and Evaluation Publicly financed programs should be accountable and demonstrate effectiveness.	**$1.18**
V. Administration and Management Complex, integrated programs require experienced staff to provide fiscal management, accountability, and coordination.	**$0.59**
Total	**$13.59**

Note: A justification for each program element and the rationale for the budget estimates are provided in Section A. The funding estimates presented are based on adjustments for changes in population and inflation since the 1999 publication. The recommended levels of investment (per capita and total) are presented in 2007 dollars using 2006 population estimates. These should be updated annually according to the U.S. Department of Labor Consumer Price Index and U.S. Census Bureau. The actual funding required for implementing programs will vary depending on state characteristics such as tobacco use prevalence, socio-demographic factors, and other factors. See Appendix E for data sources on deaths, costs, revenue and state-specific factors.

Office on Smoking and Health • Centers for Disease Control and Prevention
www.cdc.gov/tobacco • tobaccoinfo@cdc.gov • 1 (800) CDC INFO or 1 (800) 232-4636

CDC Recommended Annual Investment $53.5 million

Deaths in Louisiana Caused by Smoking

Annual average smoking-attributable deaths	6,400
Youth ages 0-17 projected to die from smoking	109,000

Annual Costs Incurred in Louisiana from Smoking

Total medical	$1,474 million
Medicaid medical	$663 million
Lost productivity from premature death	$1,919 million

State Revenue from Tobacco Excise Taxes and Settlement

FY 2006 tobacco tax revenue	$136.1 million
FY 2006 tobacco settlement payment	$131.5 million

Total state revenue from tobacco excise taxes and settlement $267.6 million

Percent tobacco revenue to fund at CDC recommended level   20%

	Per Capita Recommendation
I. State and Community Interventions Multiple societal resources working together have the greatest long-term population impact.	$5.31
II. Health Communication Interventions Media interventions prevent tobacco use initiation, promote cessation, and shape social norms.	$1.59
III. Cessation Interventions Tobacco use treatment is highly cost-effective.	$3.94
IV. Surveillance and Evaluation Publicly financed programs should be accountable and demonstrate effectiveness.	$1.08
V. Administration and Management Complex, integrated programs require experienced staff to provide fiscal management, accountability, and coordination.	$0.54
Total	**$12.46**

Note: A justification for each program element and the rationale for the budget estimates are provided in Section A. The funding estimates presented are based on adjustments for changes in population and inflation since the 1999 publication. The recommended levels of investment (per capita and total) are presented in 2007 dollars using 2006 population estimates. These should be updated annually according to the U.S. Department of Labor Consumer Price Index and U.S. Census Bureau. The actual funding required for implementing programs will vary depending on state characteristics such as tobacco use prevalence, socio-demographic factors, and other factors. See Appendix E for data sources on deaths, costs, revenue and state-specific factors.

Office on Smoking and Health • Centers for Disease Control and Prevention
www.cdc.gov/tobacco • tobaccoinfo@cdc.gov • 1 (800) CDC INFO or 1 (800) 232-4636

CDC Recommended Annual Investment $18.5 million

Deaths in Maine Caused by Smoking

Annual average smoking-attributable deaths	2,200
Youth ages 0-17 projected to die from smoking	27,000

Annual Costs Incurred in Maine from Smoking

Total medical	$602 million
Medicaid medical	$216 million
Lost productivity from premature death	$494 million

State Revenue from Tobacco Excise Taxes and Settlement

FY 2006 tobacco tax revenue	$157.0 million
FY 2006 tobacco settlement payment	$44.9 million
Total state revenue from tobacco excise taxes and settlement	$201.9 million

Percent tobacco revenue to fund at CDC recommended level   9%

	Per Capita Recommendation
I. State and Community Interventions Multiple societal resources working together have the greatest long-term population impact.	**$5.87**
II. Health Communication Interventions Media interventions prevent tobacco use initiation, promote cessation, and shape social norms.	**$2.41**
III. Cessation Interventions Tobacco use treatment is highly cost-effective.	**$3.82**
IV. Surveillance and Evaluation Publicly financed programs should be accountable and demonstrate effectiveness.	**$1.21**
V. Administration and Management Complex, integrated programs require experienced staff to provide fiscal management, accountability, and coordination.	**$0.61**
Total	**$13.92**

Note: A justification for each program element and the rationale for the budget estimates are provided in Section A. The funding estimates presented are based on adjustments for changes in population and inflation since the 1999 publication. The recommended levels of investment (per capita and total) are presented in 2007 dollars using 2006 population estimates. These should be updated annually according to the U.S. Department of Labor Consumer Price Index and U.S. Census Bureau. The actual funding required for implementing programs will vary depending on state characteristics such as tobacco use prevalence, socio-demographic factors, and other factors. See Appendix E for data sources on deaths, costs, revenue and state-specific factors.

Office on Smoking and Health • Centers for Disease Control and Prevention
www.cdc.gov/tobacco • tobaccoinfo@cdc.gov • 1 (800) CDC INFO or 1 (800) 232-4636

CDC Recommended Annual Investment $63.3 million

Deaths in Maryland Caused by Smoking

Annual average smoking-attributable deaths	6,800
Youth ages 0-17 projected to die from smoking	108,000

Annual Costs Incurred in Maryland from Smoking

Total medical	$1,964 million
Medicaid medical	$476 million
Lost productivity from premature death	$1,783 million

State Revenue from Tobacco Excise Taxes and Settlement

FY 2006 tobacco tax revenue	$279.8 million
FY 2006 tobacco settlement payment	$131.8 million

Total state revenue from tobacco excise taxes and settlement $411.6 million

Percent tobacco revenue to fund at CDC recommended level   15%

	Per Capita Recommendation
I. State and Community Interventions Multiple societal resources working together have the greatest long-term population impact.	**$4.38**
II. Health Communication Interventions Media interventions prevent tobacco use initiation, promote cessation, and shape social norms.	**$2.17**
III. Cessation Interventions Tobacco use treatment is highly cost-effective.	**$3.24**
IV. Surveillance and Evaluation Publicly financed programs should be accountable and demonstrate effectiveness.	**$0.98**
V. Administration and Management Complex, integrated programs require experienced staff to provide fiscal management, accountability, and coordination.	**$0.49**
Total	**$11.26**

Note: A justification for each program element and the rationale for the budget estimates are provided in Section A. The funding estimates presented are based on adjustments for changes in population and inflation since the 1999 publication. The recommended levels of investment (per capita and total) are presented in 2007 dollars using 2006 population estimates. These should be updated annually according to the U.S. Department of Labor Consumer Price Index and U.S. Census Bureau. The actual funding required for implementing programs will vary depending on state characteristics such as tobacco use prevalence, socio-demographic factors, and other factors. See Appendix E for data sources on deaths, costs, revenue and state-specific factors.

Office on Smoking and Health • Centers for Disease Control and Prevention
www.cdc.gov/tobacco • tobaccoinfo@cdc.gov • 1 (800) CDC INFO or 1 (800) 232-4636

CDC Recommended Annual Investment $90.0 million

Deaths in Massachusetts Caused by Smoking

Annual average smoking-attributable deaths	9,000
Youth ages 0-17 projected to die from smoking	117,000

Annual Costs Incurred in Massachusetts from Smoking

Total medical	$3,543 million
Medicaid medical	$1,046 million
Lost productivity from premature death	$1,923 million

State Revenue from Tobacco Excise Taxes and Settlement

FY 2006 tobacco tax revenue	$437.0 million
FY 2006 tobacco settlement payment	$235.6 million

Total state revenue from tobacco excise taxes and settlement $672.6 million

Percent tobacco revenue to fund at CDC recommended level   13%

	Per Capita Recommendation
I. State and Community Interventions Multiple societal resources working together have the greatest long-term population impact.	**$4.92**
II. Health Communication Interventions Media interventions prevent tobacco use initiation, promote cessation, and shape social norms.	**$3.90**
III. Cessation Interventions Tobacco use treatment is highly cost-effective.	**$3.33**
IV. Surveillance and Evaluation Publicly financed programs should be accountable and demonstrate effectiveness.	**$1.22**
V. Administration and Management Complex, integrated programs require experienced staff to provide fiscal management, accountability, and coordination.	**$0.61**
Total	**$13.98**

Note: A justification for each program element and the rationale for the budget estimates are provided in Section A. The funding estimates presented are based on adjustments for changes in population and inflation since the 1999 publication. The recommended levels of investment (per capita and total) are presented in 2007 dollars using 2006 population estimates. These should be updated annually according to the U.S. Department of Labor Consumer Price Index and U.S. Census Bureau. The actual funding required for implementing programs will vary depending on state characteristics such as tobacco use prevalence, socio-demographic factors, and other factors. See Appendix E for data sources on deaths, costs, revenue and state-specific factors.

Office on Smoking and Health • Centers for Disease Control and Prevention
www.cdc.gov/tobacco • tobaccoinfo@cdc.gov • 1 (800) CDC INFO or 1 (800) 232-4636

CDC Recommended Annual Investment $121.2 million

Deaths in Michigan Caused by Smoking

Annual average smoking-attributable deaths	14,500
Youth ages 0-17 projected to die from smoking	298,000

Annual Costs Incurred in Michigan from Smoking

Total medical	$3,401 million
Medicaid medical	$1,128 million
Lost productivity from premature death	$3,802 million

State Revenue from Tobacco Excise Taxes and Settlement

FY 2006 tobacco tax revenue	$1,166.1 million
FY 2006 tobacco settlement payment	$253.8 million
Total state revenue from tobacco excise taxes and settlement	$1,419.9 million

Percent tobacco revenue to fund at CDC recommended level   9%

	Per Capita Recommendation
I. State and Community Interventions Multiple societal resources working together have the greatest long-term population impact.	**$4.94**
II. Health Communication Interventions Media interventions prevent tobacco use initiation, promote cessation, and shape social norms.	**$1.66**
III. Cessation Interventions Tobacco use treatment is highly cost-effective.	**$3.83**
IV. Surveillance and Evaluation Publicly financed programs should be accountable and demonstrate effectiveness.	**$1.04**
V. Administration and Management Complex, integrated programs require experienced staff to provide fiscal management, accountability, and coordination.	**$0.52**
Total	**$11.99**

Note: A justification for each program element and the rationale for the budget estimates are provided in Section A. The funding estimates presented are based on adjustments for changes in population and inflation since the 1999 publication. The recommended levels of investment (per capita and total) are presented in 2007 dollars using 2006 population estimates. These should be updated annually according to the U.S. Department of Labor Consumer Price Index and U.S. Census Bureau. The actual funding required for implementing programs will vary depending on state characteristics such as tobacco use prevalence, socio-demographic factors, and other factors. See Appendix E for data sources on deaths, costs, revenue and state-specific factors.

Office on Smoking and Health • Centers for Disease Control and Prevention
www.cdc.gov/tobacco • tobaccoinfo@cdc.gov • 1 (800) CDC INFO or 1 (800) 232-4636

CDC Recommended Annual Investment $58.4 million

Deaths in Minnesota Caused by Smoking

Annual average smoking-attributable deaths	5,500
Youth ages 0-17 projected to die from smoking	118,000

Annual Costs Incurred in Minnesota from Smoking

Total medical	$2,063 million
Medicaid medical	$465 million
Lost productivity from premature death	$1,205 million

State Revenue from Tobacco Excise Taxes and Settlement

FY 2006 tobacco tax revenue	$425.7 million
FY 2006 tobacco settlement payment	$180.8 million

Total state revenue from tobacco excise taxes and settlement $606.5 million

Percent tobacco revenue to fund at CDC recommended level   10%

	Per Capita Recommendation
I. State and Community Interventions Multiple societal resources working together have the greatest long-term population impact.	**$4.77**
II. Health Communication Interventions Media interventions prevent tobacco use initiation, promote cessation, and shape social norms.	**$1.77**
III. Cessation Interventions Tobacco use treatment is highly cost-effective.	**$3.30**
IV. Surveillance and Evaluation Publicly financed programs should be accountable and demonstrate effectiveness.	**$0.98**
V. Administration and Management Complex, integrated programs require experienced staff to provide fiscal management, accountability, and coordination.	**$0.49**
Total	**$11.31**

Note: A justification for each program element and the rationale for the budget estimates are provided in Section A. The funding estimates presented are based on adjustments for changes in population and inflation since the 1999 publication. The recommended levels of investment (per capita and total) are presented in 2007 dollars using 2006 population estimates. These should be updated annually according to the U.S. Department of Labor Consumer Price Index and U.S. Census Bureau. The actual funding required for implementing programs will vary depending on state characteristics such as tobacco use prevalence, socio-demographic factors, and other factors. See Appendix E for data sources on deaths, costs, revenue and state-specific factors.

Office on Smoking and Health • Centers for Disease Control and Prevention
www.cdc.gov/tobacco • tobaccoinfo@cdc.gov • 1 (800) CDC INFO or 1 (800) 232-4636

CDC Recommended Annual Investment $39.2 million

Deaths in Mississippi Caused by Smoking

Annual average smoking-attributable deaths	4,700
Youth ages 0-17 projected to die from smoking	69,000

Annual Costs Incurred in Mississippi from Smoking

Total medical	$719 million
Medicaid medical	$264 million
Lost productivity from premature death	$1,413 million

State Revenue from Tobacco Excise Taxes and Settlement

FY 2006 tobacco tax revenue	$58.1 million
FY 2006 tobacco settlement payment	$100.5 million

Total state revenue from tobacco excise taxes and settlement $158.6 million

Percent tobacco revenue to fund at CDC recommended level   25%

	Per Capita Recommendation
I. State and Community Interventions Multiple societal resources working together have the greatest long-term population impact.	$5.44
II. Health Communication Interventions Media interventions prevent tobacco use initiation, promote cessation, and shape social norms.	$2.13
III. Cessation Interventions Tobacco use treatment is highly cost-effective.	$4.14
IV. Surveillance and Evaluation Publicly financed programs should be accountable and demonstrate effectiveness.	$1.17
V. Administration and Management Complex, integrated programs require experienced staff to provide fiscal management, accountability, and coordination.	$0.59
Total	**$13.47**

Note: *A justification for each program element and the rationale for the budget estimates are provided in Section A. The funding estimates presented are based on adjustments for changes in population and inflation since the 1999 publication. The recommended levels of investment (per capita and total) are presented in 2007 dollars using 2006 population estimates. These should be updated annually according to the U.S. Department of Labor Consumer Price Index and U.S. Census Bureau. The actual funding required for implementing programs will vary depending on state characteristics such as tobacco use prevalence, socio-demographic factors, and other factors. See Appendix E for data sources on deaths, costs, revenue and state-specific factors.*

Office on Smoking and Health • Centers for Disease Control and Prevention
www.cdc.gov/tobacco • tobaccoinfo@cdc.gov • 1 (800) CDC INFO or 1 (800) 232-4636

CDC Recommended Annual Investment $73.2 million

Deaths in Missouri Caused by Smoking

Annual average smoking-attributable deaths	9,800
Youth ages 0-17 projected to die from smoking	140,000

Annual Costs Incurred in Missouri from Smoking

Total medical	$2,137 million
Medicaid medical	$532 million
Lost productivity from premature death	$2,417 million

State Revenue from Tobacco Excise Taxes and Settlement

FY 2006 tobacco tax revenue	$111.3 million
FY 2006 tobacco settlement payment	$132.7 million

Total state revenue from tobacco excise taxes and settlement $244.0 million

Percent tobacco revenue to fund at CDC recommended level   30%

	Per Capita Recommendation
I. State and Community Interventions Multiple societal resources working together have the greatest long-term population impact.	$4.95
II. Health Communication Interventions Media interventions prevent tobacco use initiation, promote cessation, and shape social norms.	$1.99
III. Cessation Interventions Tobacco use treatment is highly cost-effective.	$3.95
IV. Surveillance and Evaluation Publicly financed programs should be accountable and demonstrate effectiveness.	$1.09
V. Administration and Management Complex, integrated programs require experienced staff to provide fiscal management, accountability, and coordination.	$0.54
Total	**$12.52**

Note: A justification for each program element and the rationale for the budget estimates are provided in Section A. The funding estimates presented are based on adjustments for changes in population and inflation since the 1999 publication. The recommended levels of investment (per capita and total) are presented in 2007 dollars using 2006 population estimates. These should be updated annually according to the U.S. Department of Labor Consumer Price Index and U.S. Census Bureau. The actual funding required for implementing programs will vary depending on state characteristics such as tobacco use prevalence, socio-demographic factors, and other factors. See Appendix E for data sources on deaths, costs, revenue and state-specific factors.

Office on Smoking and Health • Centers for Disease Control and Prevention
www.cdc.gov/tobacco • tobaccoinfo@cdc.gov • 1 (800) CDC INFO or 1 (800) 232-4636

CDC Recommended Annual Investment $13.9 million

Deaths in Montana Caused by Smoking
Annual average smoking-attributable deaths	1,400
Youth ages 0-17 projected to die from smoking	18,000

Annual Costs Incurred in Montana from Smoking
Total medical	$277 million
Medicaid medical	$67 million
Lost productivity from premature death	$295 million

State Revenue from Tobacco Excise Taxes and Settlement
FY 2006 tobacco tax revenue	$90.8 million
FY 2006 tobacco settlement payment	$24.8 million
Total state revenue from tobacco excise taxes and settlement	$115.6 million

Percent tobacco revenue to fund at CDC recommended level   12%

	Per Capita Recommendation
I. State and Community Interventions Multiple societal resources working together have the greatest long-term population impact.	$6.71
II. Health Communication Interventions Media interventions prevent tobacco use initiation, promote cessation, and shape social norms.	$2.69
III. Cessation Interventions Tobacco use treatment is effective and highly cost-effective.	$3.46
IV. Surveillance and Evaluation Publicly financed programs should be accountable and demonstrate effectiveness.	$1.29
V. Administration and Management Complex, integrated programs require experienced staff to provide fiscal management, accountability, and coordination.	$0.64
Total	**$14.79**

Note: *A justification for each program element and the rationale for the budget estimates are provided in Section A. The funding estimates presented are based on adjustments for changes in population and inflation since the 1999 publication. The recommended levels of investment (per capita and total) are presented in 2007 dollars using 2006 population estimates. These should be updated annually according to the U.S. Department of Labor Consumer Price Index and U.S. Census Bureau. The actual funding required for implementing programs will vary depending on state characteristics such as tobacco use prevalence, socio-demographic factors, and other factors. See Appendix E for data sources on deaths, costs, revenue and state-specific factors.*

Office on Smoking and Health • Centers for Disease Control and Prevention
www.cdc.gov/tobacco • tobaccoinfo@cdc.gov • 1 (800) CDC INFO or 1 (800) 232-4636

CDC Recommended Annual Investment $21.5 million

Deaths in Nebraska Caused by Smoking

Annual average smoking-attributable deaths	2,400
Youth ages 0-17 projected to die from smoking	36,000

Annual Costs Incurred in Nebraska from Smoking

Total medical	$537 million
Medicaid medical	$134 million
Lost productivity from premature death	$499 million

State Revenue from Tobacco Excise Taxes and Settlement

FY 2006 tobacco tax revenue	$71.1 million
FY 2006 tobacco settlement payment	$34.7 million
Total state revenue from tobacco excise taxes and settlement	$105.8 million

Percent tobacco revenue to fund at CDC recommended level   20%

	Per Capita Recommendation
I. State and Community Interventions Multiple societal resources working together have the greatest long-term population impact.	**$5.29**
II. Health Communication Interventions Media interventions prevent tobacco use initiation, promote cessation, and shape social norms.	**$2.00**
III. Cessation Interventions Tobacco use treatment is highly cost-effective.	**$3.32**
IV. Surveillance and Evaluation Publicly financed programs should be accountable and demonstrate effectiveness.	**$1.06**
V. Administration and Management Complex, integrated programs require experienced staff to provide fiscal management, accountability, and coordination.	**$0.53**
Total	**$12.20**

Note: A justification for each program element and the rationale for the budget estimates are provided in Section A. The funding estimates presented are based on adjustments for changes in population and inflation since the 1999 publication. The recommended levels of investment (per capita and total) are presented in 2007 dollars using 2006 population estimates. These should be updated annually according to the U.S. Department of Labor Consumer Price Index and U.S. Census Bureau. The actual funding required for implementing programs will vary depending on state characteristics such as tobacco use prevalence, socio-demographic factors, and other factors. See Appendix E for data sources on deaths, costs, revenue and state-specific factors.

Office on Smoking and Health • Centers for Disease Control and Prevention
www.cdc.gov/tobacco • tobaccoinfo@cdc.gov • 1 (800) CDC INFO or 1 (800) 232-4636

CDC Recommended Annual Investment $32.5 million

Deaths in Nevada Caused by Smoking

Annual average smoking-attributable deaths	3,100
Youth ages 0-17 projected to die from smoking	47,000

Annual Costs Incurred in Nevada from Smoking

Total medical	$565 million
Medicaid medical	$123 million
Lost productivity from premature death	$832 million

State Revenue from Tobacco Excise Taxes and Settlement

FY 2006 tobacco tax revenue	$138.2 million
FY 2006 tobacco settlement payment	$35.6 million
Total state revenue from tobacco excise taxes and settlement	$173.8 million

Percent tobacco revenue to fund at CDC recommended level   19%

	Per Capita Recommendation
I. State and Community Interventions Multiple societal resources working together have the greatest long-term population impact.	**$5.42**
II. Health Communication Interventions Media interventions prevent tobacco use initiation, promote cessation, and shape social norms.	**$2.18**
III. Cessation Interventions Tobacco use treatment is highly cost-effective.	**$3.77**
IV. Surveillance and Evaluation Publicly financed programs should be accountable and demonstrate effectiveness.	**$1.14**
V. Administration and Management Complex, integrated programs require experienced staff to provide fiscal management, accountability, and coordination.	**$0.57**
Total	**$13.08**

Note: *A justification for each program element and the rationale for the budget estimates are provided in Section A. The funding estimates presented are based on adjustments for changes in population and inflation since the 1999 publication. The recommended levels of investment (per capita and total) are presented in 2007 dollars using 2006 population estimates. These should be updated annually according to the U.S. Department of Labor Consumer Price Index and U.S. Census Bureau. The actual funding required for implementing programs will vary depending on state characteristics such as tobacco use prevalence, socio-demographic factors, and other factors. See Appendix E for data sources on deaths, costs, revenue and state-specific factors.*

Office on Smoking and Health • Centers for Disease Control and Prevention
www.cdc.gov/tobacco • tobaccoinfo@cdc.gov • 1 (800) CDC INFO or 1 (800) 232-4636

CDC Recommended Annual Investment $19.2 million

Deaths in New Hampshire Caused by Smoking

Annual average smoking-attributable deaths	1,800
Youth ages 0-17 projected to die from smoking	31,000

Annual Costs Incurred in New Hampshire from Smoking

Total medical	$564 million
Medicaid medical	$115 million
Lost productivity from premature death	$405 million

State Revenue from Tobacco Excise Taxes and Settlement

FY 2006 tobacco tax revenue	$143.4 million
FY 2006 tobacco settlement payment	$38.8 million
Total state revenue from tobacco excise taxes and settlement	$182.2 million

Percent tobacco revenue to fund at CDC recommended level   11%

	Per Capita Recommendation
I. State and Community Interventions Multiple societal resources working together have the greatest long-term population impact.	**$5.37**
II. Health Communication Interventions Media interventions prevent tobacco use initiation, promote cessation, and shape social norms.	**$3.90**
III. Cessation Interventions Tobacco use treatment is highly cost-effective.	**$3.41**
IV. Surveillance and Evaluation Publicly financed programs should be accountable and demonstrate effectiveness.	**$1.27**
V. Administration and Management Complex, integrated programs require experienced staff to provide fiscal management, accountability, and coordination.	**$0.63**
Total	**$14.58**

Note: *A justification for each program element and the rationale for the budget estimates are provided in Section A. The funding estimates presented are based on adjustments for changes in population and inflation since the 1999 publication. The recommended levels of investment (per capita and total) are presented in 2007 dollars using 2006 population estimates. These should be updated annually according to the U.S. Department of Labor Consumer Price Index and U.S. Census Bureau. The actual funding required for implementing programs will vary depending on state characteristics such as tobacco use prevalence, socio-demographic factors, and other factors. See Appendix E for data sources on deaths, costs, revenue and state-specific factors.*

Office on Smoking and Health • Centers for Disease Control and Prevention
www.cdc.gov/tobacco • tobaccoinfo@cdc.gov • 1 (800) CDC INFO or 1 (800) 232-4636

CDC Recommended Annual Investment $119.8 million

Deaths in New Jersey Caused by Smoking

Annual average smoking-attributable deaths	11,300
Youth ages 0-17 projected to die from smoking	168,000

Annual Costs Incurred in New Jersey from Smoking

Total medical	$3,178 million
Medicaid medical	$967 million
Lost productivity from premature death	$2,624 million

State Revenue from Tobacco Excise Taxes and Settlement

FY 2006 tobacco tax revenue	$802.4 million
FY 2006 tobacco settlement payment	$225.5 million
Total state revenue from tobacco excise taxes and settlement	$1,027.9 million

Percent tobacco revenue to fund at CDC recommended level   12%

	Per Capita Recommendation
I. State and Community Interventions Multiple societal resources working together have the greatest long-term population impact.	**$4.76**
II. Health Communication Interventions Media interventions prevent tobacco use initiation, promote cessation, and shape social norms.	**$3.90**
III. Cessation Interventions Tobacco use treatment is highly cost-effective.	**$3.29**
IV. Surveillance and Evaluation Publicly financed programs should be accountable and demonstrate effectiveness.	**$1.20**
V. Administration and Management Complex, integrated programs require experienced staff to provide fiscal management, accountability, and coordination.	**$0.60**
Total	**$13.75**

Note: A justification for each program element and the rationale for the budget estimates are provided in Section A. The funding estimates presented are based on adjustments for changes in population and inflation since the 1999 publication. The recommended levels of investment (per capita and total) are presented in 2007 dollars using 2006 population estimates. These should be updated annually according to the U.S. Department of Labor Consumer Price Index and U.S. Census Bureau. The actual funding required for implementing programs will vary depending on state characteristics such as tobacco use prevalence, socio-demographic factors, and other factors. See Appendix E for data sources on deaths, costs, revenue and state-specific factors.

Office on Smoking and Health • Centers for Disease Control and Prevention
www.cdc.gov/tobacco • tobaccoinfo@cdc.gov • 1 (800) CDC INFO or 1 (800) 232-4636

CDC Recommended Annual Investment $23.4 million

Deaths in New Mexico Caused by Smoking

Annual average smoking-attributable deaths	2,100
Youth ages 0-17 projected to die from smoking	38,000

Annual Costs Incurred in New Mexico from Smoking

Total medical	$461 million
Medicaid medical	$184 million
Lost productivity from premature death	$467 million

State Revenue from Tobacco Excise Taxes and Settlement

FY 2006 tobacco tax revenue	$65.8 million
FY 2006 tobacco settlement payment	$34.8 million

Total state revenue from tobacco excise taxes and settlement $100.6 million

Percent tobacco revenue to fund at CDC recommended level   23%

	Per Capita Recommendation
I. State and Community Interventions Multiple societal resources working together have the greatest long-term population impact.	**$5.55**
II. Health Communication Interventions Media interventions prevent tobacco use initiation, promote cessation, and shape social norms.	**$1.33**
III. Cessation Interventions Tobacco use treatment is highly cost-effective.	**$3.51**
IV. Surveillance and Evaluation Publicly financed programs should be accountable and demonstrate effectiveness.	**$1.04**
V. Administration and Management Complex, integrated programs require experienced staff to provide fiscal management, accountability, and coordination.	**$0.52**
Total	**$11.95**

Note: A justification for each program element and the rationale for the budget estimates are provided in Section A. The funding estimates presented are based on adjustments for changes in population and inflation since the 1999 publication. The recommended levels of investment (per capita and total) are presented in 2007 dollars using 2006 population estimates. These should be updated annually according to the U.S. Department of Labor Consumer Price Index and U.S. Census Bureau. The actual funding required for implementing programs will vary depending on state characteristics such as tobacco use prevalence, socio-demographic factors, and other factors. See Appendix E for data sources on deaths, costs, revenue and state-specific factors.

Office on Smoking and Health • Centers for Disease Control and Prevention
www.cdc.gov/tobacco • tobaccoinfo@cdc.gov • 1 (800) CDC INFO or 1 (800) 232-4636

CDC Recommended Annual Investment $254.3 million

Deaths in New York Caused by Smoking

Annual average smoking-attributable deaths	25,500
Youth ages 0-17 projected to die from smoking	389,000

Annual Costs Incurred in New York from Smoking

Total medical	$8,171 million
Medicaid medical	$5,471 million
Lost productivity from premature death	$6,018 million

State Revenue from Tobacco Excise Taxes and Settlement

FY 2006 tobacco tax revenue	$981.0 million
FY 2006 tobacco settlement payment	$744.4 million
Total state revenue from tobacco excise taxes and settlement	$1,725.4 million

Percent tobacco revenue to fund at CDC recommended level   15%

	Per Capita Recommendation
I. State and Community Interventions Multiple societal resources working together have the greatest long-term population impact.	**$4.65**
II. Health Communication Interventions Media interventions prevent tobacco use initiation, promote cessation, and shape social norms.	**$3.42**
III. Cessation Interventions Tobacco use treatment is highly cost-effective.	**$3.37**
IV. Surveillance and Evaluation Publicly financed programs should be accountable and demonstrate effectiveness.	**$1.14**
V. Administration and Management Complex, integrated programs require experienced staff to provide fiscal management, accountability, and coordination.	**$0.57**
Total	**$13.15**

Note: A justification for each program element and the rationale for the budget estimates are provided in Section A. The funding estimates presented are based on adjustments for changes in population and inflation since the 1999 publication. The recommended levels of investment (per capita and total) are presented in 2007 dollars using 2006 population estimates. These should be updated annually according to the U.S. Department of Labor Consumer Price Index and U.S. Census Bureau. The actual funding required for implementing programs will vary depending on state characteristics such as tobacco use prevalence, socio-demographic factors, and other factors. See Appendix E for data sources on deaths, costs, revenue and state-specific factors.

Office on Smoking and Health • Centers for Disease Control and Prevention
www.cdc.gov/tobacco • tobaccoinfo@cdc.gov • 1 (800) CDC INFO or 1 (800) 232-4636

CDC Recommended Annual Investment $106.8 million

Deaths in North Carolina Caused by Smoking

Annual average smoking-attributable deaths	11,900
Youth ages 0-17 projected to die from smoking	193,000

Annual Costs Incurred in North Carolina from Smoking

Total medical	$2,463 million
Medicaid medical	$769 million
Lost productivity from premature death	$3,307 million

State Revenue from Tobacco Excise Taxes and Settlement

FY 2006 tobacco tax revenue	$172.3 million
FY 2006 tobacco settlement payment	$136.0 million

Total state revenue from tobacco excise taxes and settlement $308.3 million

Percent tobacco revenue to fund at CDC recommended level   35%

	Per Capita Recommendation
I. State and Community Interventions Multiple societal resources working together have the greatest long-term population impact.	**$4.84**
II. Health Communication Interventions Media interventions prevent tobacco use initiation, promote cessation, and shape social norms.	**$1.83**
III. Cessation Interventions Tobacco use treatment is highly cost-effective.	**$3.82**
IV. Surveillance and Evaluation Publicly financed programs should be accountable and demonstrate effectiveness.	**$1.05**
V. Administration and Management Complex, integrated programs require experienced staff to provide fiscal management, accountability, and coordination.	**$0.52**
Total	**$12.06**

Note: A justification for each program element and the rationale for the budget estimates are provided in Section A. The funding estimates presented are based on adjustments for changes in population and inflation since the 1999 publication. The recommended levels of investment (per capita and total) are presented in 2007 dollars using 2006 population estimates. These should be updated annually according to the U.S. Department of Labor Consumer Price Index and U.S. Census Bureau. The actual funding required for implementing programs will vary depending on state characteristics such as tobacco use prevalence, socio-demographic factors, and other factors. See Appendix E for data sources on deaths, costs, revenue and state-specific factors.

Office on Smoking and Health • Centers for Disease Control and Prevention
www.cdc.gov/tobacco • tobaccoinfo@cdc.gov • 1 (800) CDC INFO or 1 (800) 232-4636

North Dakota

CDC Recommended Annual Investment $9.3 million

Deaths in North Dakota Caused by Smoking

Annual average smoking-attributable deaths	900
Youth ages 0-17 projected to die from smoking	11,000

Annual Costs Incurred in North Dakota from Smoking

Total medical	$247 million
Medicaid medical	$47 million
Lost productivity from premature death	$190 million

State Revenue from Tobacco Excise Taxes and Settlement

FY 2006 tobacco tax revenue	$23.3 million
FY 2006 tobacco settlement payment	$21.3 million
Total state revenue from tobacco excise taxes and settlement	$44.6 million

Percent tobacco revenue to fund at CDC recommended level   21%

	Per Capita Recommendation
I. State and Community Interventions Multiple societal resources working together have the greatest long-term population impact.	$7.37
II. Health Communication Interventions Media interventions prevent tobacco use initiation, promote cessation, and shape social norms.	$1.86
III. Cessation Interventions Tobacco use treatment is highly cost-effective.	$3.52
IV. Surveillance and Evaluation Publicly financed programs should be accountable and demonstrate effectiveness.	$1.28
V. Administration and Management Complex, integrated programs require experienced staff to provide fiscal management, accountability, and coordination.	$0.64
Total	**$14.67**

Note: A justification for each program element and the rationale for the budget estimates are provided in Section A. The funding estimates presented are based on adjustments for changes in population and inflation since the 1999 publication. The recommended levels of investment (per capita and total) are presented in 2007 dollars using 2006 population estimates. These should be updated annually according to the U.S. Department of Labor Consumer Price Index and U.S. Census Bureau. The actual funding required for implementing programs will vary depending on state characteristics such as tobacco use prevalence, socio-demographic factors, and other factors. See Appendix E for data sources on deaths, costs, revenue and state-specific factors.

Office on Smoking and Health • Centers for Disease Control and Prevention
www.cdc.gov/tobacco • tobaccoinfo@cdc.gov • 1 (800) CDC INFO or 1 (800) 232-4636

CDC Recommended Annual Investment $145.0 million

Deaths in Ohio Caused by Smoking

Annual average smoking-attributable deaths	18,600
Youth ages 0-17 projected to die from smoking	293,000

Annual Costs Incurred in Ohio from Smoking

Total medical	$4,375 million
Medicaid medical	$1,426 million
Lost productivity from premature death	$4,658 million

State Revenue from Tobacco Excise Taxes and Settlement

FY 2006 tobacco tax revenue	$1,022.1 million
FY 2006 tobacco settlement payment	$293.8 million
Total state revenue from tobacco excise taxes and settlement	$1,315.9 million

Percent tobacco revenue to fund at CDC recommended level   11%

		Per Capita Recommendation
I.	**State and Community Interventions** Multiple societal resources working together have the greatest long-term population impact.	**$5.12**
II.	**Health Communication Interventions** Media interventions prevent tobacco use initiation, promote cessation, and shape social norms.	**$2.02**
III.	**Cessation Interventions** Tobacco use treatment is highly cost-effective.	**$3.85**
IV.	**Surveillance and Evaluation** Publicly financed programs should be accountable and demonstrate effectiveness.	**$1.10**
V.	**Administration and Management** Complex, integrated programs require experienced staff to provide fiscal management, accountability, and coordination.	**$0.55**
	Total	**$12.64**

Note: A justification for each program element and the rationale for the budget estimates are provided in Section A. The funding estimates presented are based on adjustments for changes in population and inflation since the 1999 publication. The recommended levels of investment (per capita and total) are presented in 2007 dollars using 2006 population estimates. These should be updated annually according to the U.S. Department of Labor Consumer Price Index and U.S. Census Bureau. The actual funding required for implementing programs will vary depending on state characteristics such as tobacco use prevalence, socio-demographic factors, and other factors. See Appendix E for data sources on deaths, costs, revenue and state-specific factors.

Office on Smoking and Health • Centers for Disease Control and Prevention
www.cdc.gov/tobacco • tobaccoinfo@cdc.gov • 1 (800) CDC INFO or 1 (800) 232-4636

CDC Recommended Annual Investment $45.0 million

Deaths in Oklahoma Caused by Smoking

Annual average smoking-attributable deaths	5,800
Youth ages 0-17 projected to die from smoking	87,000

Annual Costs Incurred in Oklahoma from Smoking

Total medical	$1,162 million
Medicaid medical	$218 million
Lost productivity from premature death	$1,556 million

State Revenue from Tobacco Excise Taxes and Settlement

FY 2006 tobacco tax revenue	$224.4 million
FY 2006 tobacco settlement payment	$60.4 million

Total state revenue from tobacco excise taxes and settlement $284.8 million

Percent tobacco revenue to fund at CDC recommended level   16%

	Per Capita Recommendation
I. State and Community Interventions Multiple societal resources working together have the greatest long-term population impact.	**$5.38**
II. Health Communication Interventions Media interventions prevent tobacco use initiation, promote cessation, and shape social norms.	**$1.34**
III. Cessation Interventions Tobacco use treatment is highly cost-effective.	**$4.18**
IV. Surveillance and Evaluation Publicly financed programs should be accountable and demonstrate effectiveness.	**$1.09**
V. Administration and Management Complex, integrated programs require experienced staff to provide fiscal management, accountability, and coordination.	**$0.55**
Total	**$12.54**

Note: A justification for each program element and the rationale for the budget estimates are provided in Section A. The funding estimates presented are based on adjustments for changes in population and inflation since the 1999 publication. The recommended levels of investment (per capita and total) are presented in 2007 dollars using 2006 population estimates. These should be updated annually according to the U.S. Department of Labor Consumer Price Index and U.S. Census Bureau. The actual funding required for implementing programs will vary depending on state characteristics such as tobacco use prevalence, socio-demographic factors, and other factors. See Appendix E for data sources on deaths, costs, revenue and state-specific factors.

Office on Smoking and Health • Centers for Disease Control and Prevention
www.cdc.gov/tobacco • tobaccoinfo@cdc.gov • 1 (800) CDC INFO or 1 (800) 232-4636

CDC Recommended Annual Investment $43.0 million

Deaths in Oregon Caused by Smoking

Annual average smoking-attributable deaths	5,000
Youth ages 0-17 projected to die from smoking	74,000

Annual Costs Incurred in Oregon from Smoking

Total medical	$1,116 million
Medicaid medical	$287 million
Lost productivity from premature death	$1,077 million

State Revenue from Tobacco Excise Taxes and Settlement

FY 2006 tobacco tax revenue	$263.9 million
FY 2006 tobacco settlement payment	$66.9 million

Total state revenue from tobacco excise taxes and settlement $330.8 million

Percent tobacco revenue to fund at CDC recommended level   13%

		Per Capita Recommendation
I.	**State and Community Interventions** Multiple societal resources working together have the greatest long-term population impact.	$4.80
II.	**Health Communication Interventions** Media interventions prevent tobacco use initiation, promote cessation, and shape social norms.	$1.88
III.	**Cessation Interventions** Tobacco use treatment is highly cost-effective.	$3.41
IV.	**Surveillance and Evaluation** Publicly financed programs should be accountable and demonstrate effectiveness.	$1.01
V.	**Administration and Management** Complex, integrated programs require experienced staff to provide fiscal management, accountability, and coordination.	$0.50
	Total	**$11.60**

Note: A justification for each program element and the rationale for the budget estimates are provided in Section A. The funding estimates presented are based on adjustments for changes in population and inflation since the 1999 publication. The recommended levels of investment (per capita and total) are presented in 2007 dollars using 2006 population estimates. These should be updated annually according to the U.S. Department of Labor Consumer Price Index and U.S. Census Bureau. The actual funding required for implementing programs will vary depending on state characteristics such as tobacco use prevalence, socio-demographic factors, and other factors. See Appendix E for data sources on deaths, costs, revenue and state-specific factors.

Office on Smoking and Health • Centers for Disease Control and Prevention
www.cdc.gov/tobacco • tobaccoinfo@cdc.gov • 1 (800) CDC INFO or 1 (800) 232-4636

CDC Recommended Annual Investment $155.5 million

Deaths in Pennsylvania Caused by Smoking

Annual average smoking-attributable deaths	20,100
Youth ages 0-17 projected to die from smoking	300,000

Annual Costs Incurred in Pennsylvania from Smoking

Total medical	$5,193 million
Medicaid medical	$1,710 million
Lost productivity from premature death	$4,637 million

State Revenue from Tobacco Excise Taxes and Settlement

FY 2006 tobacco tax revenue	$1,034.0 million
FY 2006 tobacco settlement payment	$335.2 million
Total state revenue from tobacco excise taxes and settlement	$1,369.2 million

Percent tobacco revenue to fund at CDC recommended level   11%

	Per Capita Recommendation
I. State and Community Interventions Multiple societal resources working together have the greatest long-term population impact.	$4.49
II. Health Communication Interventions Media interventions prevent tobacco use initiation, promote cessation, and shape social norms.	$2.57
III. Cessation Interventions Tobacco use treatment is highly cost-effective.	$3.80
IV. Surveillance and Evaluation Publicly financed programs should be accountable and demonstrate effectiveness.	$1.09
V. Administration and Management Complex, integrated programs require experienced staff to provide fiscal management, accountability, and coordination.	$0.54
Total	**$12.49**

Note: *A justification for each program element and the rationale for the budget estimates are provided in Section A. The funding estimates presented are based on adjustments for changes in population and inflation since the 1999 publication. The recommended levels of investment (per capita and total) are presented in 2007 dollars using 2006 population estimates. These should be updated annually according to the U.S. Department of Labor Consumer Price Index and U.S. Census Bureau. The actual funding required for implementing programs will vary depending on state characteristics such as tobacco use prevalence, socio-demographic factors, and other factors. See Appendix E for data sources on deaths, costs, revenue and state-specific factors.*

Office on Smoking and Health • Centers for Disease Control and Prevention
www.cdc.gov/tobacco • tobaccoinfo@cdc.gov • 1 (800) CDC INFO or 1 (800) 232-4636

CDC Recommended Annual Investment $15.2 million

Deaths in Rhode Island Caused by Smoking

Annual average smoking-attributable deaths	1,700
Youth ages 0-17 projected to die from smoking	23,000

Annual Costs Incurred in Rhode Island from Smoking

Total medical	$506 million
Medicaid medical	$179 million
Lost productivity from premature death	$364 million

State Revenue from Tobacco Excise Taxes and Settlement

FY 2006 tobacco tax revenue	$125.9 million
FY 2006 tobacco settlement payment	$41.9 million
Total state revenue from tobacco excise taxes and settlement	$167.8 million

Percent tobacco revenue to fund at CDC recommended level   9%

	Per Capita Recommendation
I. State and Community Interventions Multiple societal resources working together have the greatest long-term population impact.	**$6.28**
II. Health Communication Interventions Media interventions prevent tobacco use initiation, promote cessation, and shape social norms.	**$2.53**
III. Cessation Interventions Tobacco use treatment is highly cost-effective.	**$3.54**
IV. Surveillance and Evaluation Publicly financed programs should be accountable and demonstrate effectiveness.	**$1.24**
V. Administration and Management Complex, integrated programs require experienced staff to provide fiscal management, accountability, and coordination.	**$0.62**
Total	**$14.21**

Note: A justification for each program element and the rationale for the budget estimates are provided in Section A. The funding estimates presented are based on adjustments for changes in population and inflation since the 1999 publication. The recommended levels of investment (per capita and total) are presented in 2007 dollars using 2006 population estimates. These should be updated annually according to the U.S. Department of Labor Consumer Price Index and U.S. Census Bureau. The actual funding required for implementing programs will vary depending on state characteristics such as tobacco use prevalence, socio-demographic factors, and other factors. See Appendix E for data sources on deaths, costs, revenue and state-specific factors.

Office on Smoking and Health • Centers for Disease Control and Prevention
www.cdc.gov/tobacco • tobaccoinfo@cdc.gov • 1 (800) CDC INFO or 1 (800) 232-4636

CDC Recommended Annual Investment $62.2 million

Deaths in South Carolina Caused by Smoking

Annual average smoking-attributable deaths	5,900
Youth ages 0-17 projected to die from smoking	103,000

Annual Costs Incurred in South Carolina from Smoking

Total medical	$1,095 million
Medicaid medical	$393 million
Lost productivity from premature death	$1,835 million

State Revenue from Tobacco Excise Taxes and Settlement

FY 2006 tobacco tax revenue	$32.4 million
FY 2006 tobacco settlement payment	$68.6 million

Total state revenue from tobacco excise taxes and settlement $101.0 million

Percent tobacco revenue to fund at CDC recommended level   62%

	Per Capita Recommendation
I. State and Community Interventions Multiple societal resources working together have the greatest long-term population impact.	$4.74
II. Health Communication Interventions Media interventions prevent tobacco use initiation, promote cessation, and shape social norms.	$3.90
III. Cessation Interventions Tobacco use treatment is highly cost-effective.	$3.87
IV. Surveillance and Evaluation Publicly financed programs should be accountable and demonstrate effectiveness.	$1.25
V. Administration and Management Complex, integrated programs require experienced staff to provide fiscal management, accountability, and coordination.	$0.63
Total	**$14.39**

Note: A justification for each program element and the rationale for the budget estimates are provided in Section A. The funding estimates presented are based on adjustments for changes in population and inflation since the 1999 publication. The recommended levels of investment (per capita and total) are presented in 2007 dollars using 2006 population estimates. These should be updated annually according to the U.S. Department of Labor Consumer Price Index and U.S. Census Bureau. The actual funding required for implementing programs will vary depending on state characteristics such as tobacco use prevalence, socio-demographic factors, and other factors. See Appendix E for data sources on deaths, costs, revenue and state-specific factors.

Office on Smoking and Health • Centers for Disease Control and Prevention
www.cdc.gov/tobacco • tobaccoinfo@cdc.gov • 1 (800) CDC INFO or 1 (800) 232-4636

CDC Recommended Annual Investment $11.3 million

Deaths in South Dakota Caused by Smoking

Annual average smoking-attributable deaths	1,100
Youth ages 0-17 projected to die from smoking	18,000

Annual Costs Incurred in South Dakota from Smoking

Total medical	$274 million
Medicaid medical	$58 million
Lost productivity from premature death	$228 million

State Revenue from Tobacco Excise Taxes and Settlement

FY 2006 tobacco tax revenue	$28.2 million
FY 2006 tobacco settlement payment	$20.4 million
Total state revenue from tobacco excise taxes and settlement	$48.6 million

Percent tobacco revenue to fund at CDC recommended level   23%

		Per Capita Recommendation
I.	**State and Community Interventions** Multiple societal resources working together have the greatest long-term population impact.	**$7.05**
II.	**Health Communication Interventions** Media interventions prevent tobacco use initiation, promote cessation, and shape social norms.	**$1.97**
III.	**Cessation Interventions** Tobacco use treatment is highly cost-effective.	**$3.53**
IV.	**Surveillance and Evaluation** Publicly financed programs should be accountable and demonstrate effectiveness.	**$1.26**
V.	**Administration and Management** Complex, integrated programs require experienced staff to provide fiscal management, accountability, and coordination.	**$0.63**
	Total	**$14.44**

Note: A justification for each program element and the rationale for the budget estimates are provided in Section A. The funding estimates presented are based on adjustments for changes in population and inflation since the 1999 publication. The recommended levels of investment (per capita and total) are presented in 2007 dollars using 2006 population estimates. These should be updated annually according to the U.S. Department of Labor Consumer Price Index and U.S. Census Bureau. The actual funding required for implementing programs will vary depending on state characteristics such as tobacco use prevalence, socio-demographic factors, and other factors. See Appendix E for data sources on deaths, costs, revenue and state-specific factors.

Office on Smoking and Health • Centers for Disease Control and Prevention
www.cdc.gov/tobacco • tobaccoinfo@cdc.gov • 1 (800) CDC INFO or 1 (800) 232-4636

CDC Recommended Annual Investment $71.7 million

Deaths in Tennessee Caused by Smoking

Annual average smoking-attributable deaths	9,500
Youth ages 0-17 projected to die from smoking	132,000

Annual Costs Incurred in Tennessee from Smoking

Total medical	$2,166 million
Medicaid medical	$680 million
Lost productivity from premature death	$2,740 million

State Revenue from Tobacco Excise Taxes and Settlement

FY 2006 tobacco tax revenue	$124.5 million
FY 2006 tobacco settlement payment	$142.4 million

Total state revenue from tobacco excise taxes and settlement $266.9 million

Percent tobacco revenue to fund at CDC recommended level   27%

	Per Capita Recommendation
I. State and Community Interventions Multiple societal resources working together have the greatest long-term population impact.	**$4.67**
II. Health Communication Interventions Media interventions prevent tobacco use initiation, promote cessation, and shape social norms.	**$1.75**
III. Cessation Interventions Tobacco use treatment is highly cost-effective.	**$3.92**
IV. Surveillance and Evaluation Publicly financed programs should be accountable and demonstrate effectiveness.	**$1.03**
V. Administration and Management Complex, integrated programs require experienced staff to provide fiscal management, accountability, and coordination.	**$0.52**
Total	**$11.89**

Note: *A justification for each program element and the rationale for the budget estimates are provided in Section A. The funding estimates presented are based on adjustments for changes in population and inflation since the 1999 publication. The recommended levels of investment (per capita and total) are presented in 2007 dollars using 2006 population estimates. These should be updated annually according to the U.S. Department of Labor Consumer Price Index and U.S. Census Bureau. The actual funding required for implementing programs will vary depending on state characteristics such as tobacco use prevalence, socio-demographic factors, and other factors. See Appendix E for data sources on deaths, costs, revenue and state-specific factors.*

Office on Smoking and Health • Centers for Disease Control and Prevention
www.cdc.gov/tobacco • tobaccoinfo@cdc.gov • 1 (800) CDC INFO or 1 (800) 232-4636

CDC Recommended Annual Investment $266.3 million

Deaths in Texas Caused by Smoking

Annual average smoking-attributable deaths	24,200
Youth ages 0-17 projected to die from smoking	503,000

Annual Costs Incurred in Texas from Smoking

Total medical	$5,831 million
Medicaid medical	$1,620 million
Lost productivity from premature death	$6,445 million

State Revenue from Tobacco Excise Taxes and Settlement

FY 2006 tobacco tax revenue	$570.2 million
FY 2006 tobacco settlement payment	$512.6 million
Total state revenue from tobacco excise taxes and settlement	$1,082.8 million

Percent tobacco revenue to fund at CDC recommended level   25%

	Per Capita Recommendation
I. State and Community Interventions Multiple societal resources working together have the greatest long-term population impact.	**$4.85**
II. Health Communication Interventions Media interventions prevent tobacco use initiation, promote cessation, and shape social norms.	**$1.83**
III. Cessation Interventions Tobacco use treatment is highly cost-effective.	**$3.16**
IV. Surveillance and Evaluation Publicly financed programs should be accountable and demonstrate effectiveness.	**$0.98**
V. Administration and Management Complex, integrated programs require experienced staff to provide fiscal management, accountability, and coordination.	**$0.49**
Total	**$11.31**

Note: A justification for each program element and the rationale for the budget estimates are provided in Section A. The funding estimates presented are based on adjustments for changes in population and inflation since the 1999 publication. The recommended levels of investment (per capita and total) are presented in 2007 dollars using 2006 population estimates. These should be updated annually according to the U.S. Department of Labor Consumer Price Index and U.S. Census Bureau. The actual funding required for implementing programs will vary depending on state characteristics such as tobacco use prevalence, socio-demographic factors, and other factors. See Appendix E for data sources on deaths, costs, revenue and state-specific factors.

Office on Smoking and Health • Centers for Disease Control and Prevention
www.cdc.gov/tobacco • tobaccoinfo@cdc.gov • 1 (800) CDC INFO or 1 (800) 232-4636

CDC Recommended Annual Investment $23.6 million

Deaths in Utah Caused by Smoking

Annual average smoking-attributable deaths	1,100
Youth ages 0-17 projected to die from smoking	26,000

Annual Costs Incurred in Utah from Smoking

Total medical	$345 million
Medicaid medical	$104 million
Lost productivity from premature death	$273 million

State Revenue from Tobacco Excise Taxes and Settlement

FY 2006 tobacco tax revenue	$64.7 million
FY 2006 tobacco settlement payment	$25.9 million
Total state revenue from tobacco excise taxes and settlement	$90.6 million

Percent tobacco revenue to fund at CDC recommended level   26%

	Per Capita Recommendation
I. State and Community Interventions Multiple societal resources working together have the greatest long-term population impact.	**$4.55**
II. Health Communication Interventions Media interventions prevent tobacco use initiation, promote cessation, and shape social norms.	**$1.44**
III. Cessation Interventions Tobacco use treatment is highly cost-effective.	**$2.04**
IV. Surveillance and Evaluation Publicly financed programs should be accountable and demonstrate effectiveness.	**$0.80**
V. Administration and Management Complex, integrated programs require experienced staff to provide fiscal management, accountability, and coordination.	**$0.40**
Total	**$9.23**

Note: A justification for each program element and the rationale for the budget estimates are provided in Section A. The funding estimates presented are based on adjustments for changes in population and inflation since the 1999 publication. The recommended levels of investment (per capita and total) are presented in 2007 dollars using 2006 population estimates. These should be updated annually according to the U.S. Department of Labor Consumer Price Index and U.S. Census Bureau. The actual funding required for implementing programs will vary depending on state characteristics such as tobacco use prevalence, socio-demographic factors, and other factors. See Appendix E for data sources on deaths, costs, revenue and state-specific factors.

Office on Smoking and Health • Centers for Disease Control and Prevention
www.cdc.gov/tobacco • tobaccoinfo@cdc.gov • 1 (800) CDC INFO or 1 (800) 232-4636

CDC Recommended Annual Investment $10.4 million

Deaths in Vermont Caused by Smoking

Annual average smoking-attributable deaths	900
Youth ages 0-17 projected to die from smoking	12,000

Annual Costs Incurred in Vermont from Smoking

Total medical	$233 million
Medicaid medical	$72 million
Lost productivity from premature death	$197 million

State Revenue from Tobacco Excise Taxes and Settlement

FY 2006 tobacco tax revenue	$48.9 million
FY 2006 tobacco settlement payment	$24.0 million
Total state revenue from tobacco excise taxes and settlement	$72.9 million

Percent tobacco revenue to fund at CDC recommended level   14%

	Per Capita Recommendation
I. State and Community Interventions Multiple societal resources working together have the greatest long-term population impact.	$7.39
II. Health Communication Interventions Media interventions prevent tobacco use initiation, promote cessation, and shape social norms.	$3.74
III. Cessation Interventions Tobacco use treatment is highly cost-effective.	$3.43
IV. Surveillance and Evaluation Publicly financed programs should be accountable and demonstrate effectiveness.	$1.46
V. Administration and Management Complex, integrated programs require experienced staff to provide fiscal management, accountability, and coordination.	$0.73
Total	**$16.75**

Note: A justification for each program element and the rationale for the budget estimates are provided in Section A. The funding estimates presented are based on adjustments for changes in population and inflation since the 1999 publication. The recommended levels of investment (per capita and total) are presented in 2007 dollars using 2006 population estimates. These should be updated annually according to the U.S. Department of Labor Consumer Price Index and U.S. Census Bureau. The actual funding required for implementing programs will vary depending on state characteristics such as tobacco use prevalence, socio-demographic factors, and other factors. See Appendix E for data sources on deaths, costs, revenue and state-specific factors.

Office on Smoking and Health • Centers for Disease Control and Prevention
www.cdc.gov/tobacco • tobaccoinfo@cdc.gov • 1 (800) CDC INFO or 1 (800) 232-4636

CDC Recommended Annual Investment $103.2 million

Deaths in Virginia Caused by Smoking

Annual average smoking-attributable deaths	9,300
Youth ages 0 -17 projected to die from smoking	152,000

Annual Costs Incurred in Virginia from Smoking

Total medical	$2,087 million
Medicaid medical	$401 million
Lost productivity from premature death	$2,427 million

State Revenue from Tobacco Excise Taxes and Settlement

FY 2006 tobacco tax revenue	$187.1 million
FY 2006 tobacco settlement payment	$119.3 million

Total state revenue from tobacco excise taxes and settlement $306.4 million

Percent tobacco revenue to fund at CDC recommended level   34%

	Per Capita Recommendation
I. State and Community Interventions Multiple societal resources working together have the greatest long-term population impact.	$4.37
II. Health Communication Interventions Media interventions prevent tobacco use initiation, promote cessation, and shape social norms.	$3.90
III. Cessation Interventions Tobacco use treatment is highly cost-effective.	$3.47
IV. Surveillance and Evaluation Publicly financed programs should be accountable and demonstrate effectiveness.	$1.17
V. Administration and Management Complex, integrated programs require experienced staff to provide fiscal management, accountability, and coordination.	$0.59
Total	**$13.50**

Note: A justification for each program element and the rationale for the budget estimates are provided in Section A. The funding estimates presented are based on adjustments for changes in population and inflation since the 1999 publication. The recommended levels of investment (per capita and total) are presented in 2007 dollars using 2006 population estimates. These should be updated annually according to the U.S. Department of Labor Consumer Price Index and U.S. Census Bureau. The actual funding required for implementing programs will vary depending on state characteristics such as tobacco use prevalence, socio-demographic factors, and other factors. See Appendix E for data sources on deaths, costs, revenue and state-specific factors.

Office on Smoking and Health • Centers for Disease Control and Prevention
www.cdc.gov/tobacco • tobaccoinfo@cdc.gov • 1 (800) CDC INFO or 1 (800) 232-4636

CDC Recommended Annual Investment $67.3 million

Deaths in Washington Caused by Smoking

Annual average smoking-attributable deaths	7,600
Youth ages 0-17 projected to die from smoking	124,000

Annual Costs Incurred in Washington from Smoking

Total medical	$1,957 million
Medicaid medical	$651 million
Lost productivity from premature death	$1,743 million

State Revenue from Tobacco Excise Taxes and Settlement

FY 2006 tobacco tax revenue	$453.3 million
FY 2006 tobacco settlement payment	$119.8 million

Total state revenue from tobacco excise taxes and settlement $573.1 million

Percent tobacco revenue to fund at CDC recommended level   12%

	Per Capita Recommendation
I. State and Community Interventions Multiple societal resources working together have the greatest long-term population impact.	**$4.51**
II. Health Communication Interventions Media interventions prevent tobacco use initiation, promote cessation, and shape social norms.	**$1.44**
III. Cessation Interventions Tobacco use treatment is highly cost-effective.	**$3.18**
IV. Surveillance and Evaluation Publicly financed programs should be accountable and demonstrate effectiveness.	**$0.91**
V. Administration and Management Complex, integrated programs require experienced staff to provide fiscal management, accountability, and coordination.	**$0.46**
Total	**$10.50**

Note: *A justification for each program element and the rationale for the budget estimates are provided in Section A. The funding estimates presented are based on adjustments for changes in population and inflation since the 1999 publication. The recommended levels of investment (per capita and total) are presented in 2007 dollars using 2006 population estimates. These should be updated annually according to the U.S. Department of Labor Consumer Price Index and U.S. Census Bureau. The actual funding required for implementing programs will vary depending on state characteristics such as tobacco use prevalence, socio-demographic factors, and other factors. See Appendix E for data sources on deaths, costs, revenue and state-specific factors.*

Office on Smoking and Health • Centers for Disease Control and Prevention
www.cdc.gov/tobacco • tobaccoinfo@cdc.gov • 1 (800) CDC INFO or 1 (800) 232-4636

CDC Recommended Annual Investment $27.8 million

Deaths in West Virginia Caused by Smoking

Annual average smoking-attributable deaths	3,900
Youth ages 0-17 projected to die from smoking	46,000

Annual Costs Incurred in West Virginia from Smoking

Total medical	$690 million
Medicaid medical	$229 million
Lost productivity from premature death	$993 million

State Revenue from Tobacco Excise Taxes and Settlement

FY 2006 tobacco tax revenue	$112.5 million
FY 2006 tobacco settlement payment	$51.7 million

Total state revenue from tobacco excise taxes and settlement $164.2 million

Percent tobacco revenue to fund at CDC recommended level   17%

	Per Capita Recommendation
I. State and Community Interventions Multiple societal resources working together have the greatest long-term population impact.	**$5.74**
II. Health Communication Interventions Media interventions prevent tobacco use initiation, promote cessation, and shape social norms.	**$3.13**
III. Cessation Interventions Tobacco use treatment is highly cost-effective.	**$4.46**
IV. Surveillance and Evaluation Publicly financed programs should be accountable and demonstrate effectiveness.	**$1.33**
V. Administration and Management Complex, integrated programs require experienced staff to provide fiscal management, accountability, and coordination.	**$0.67**
Total	**$15.33**

Note: *A justification for each program element and the rationale for the budget estimates are provided in Section A. The funding estimates presented are based on adjustments for changes in population and inflation since the 1999 publication. The recommended levels of investment (per capita and total) are presented in 2007 dollars using 2006 population estimates. These should be updated annually according to the U.S. Department of Labor Consumer Price Index and U.S. Census Bureau. The actual funding required for implementing programs will vary depending on state characteristics such as tobacco use prevalence, socio-demographic factors, and other factors. See Appendix E for data sources on deaths, costs, revenue and state-specific factors.*

Office on Smoking and Health • Centers for Disease Control and Prevention
www.cdc.gov/tobacco • tobaccoinfo@cdc.gov • 1 (800) CDC INFO or 1 (800) 232-4636

CDC Recommended Annual Investment $64.3 million

Deaths in Wisconsin Caused by Smoking

Annual average smoking-attributable deaths	7,300
Youth ages 0-17 projected to die from smoking	128,000

Annual Costs Incurred in Wisconsin from Smoking

Total medical	$2,024 million
Medicaid medical	$480 million
Lost productivity from premature death	$1,642 million

State Revenue from Tobacco Excise Taxes and Settlement

FY 2006 tobacco tax revenue	$317.9 million
FY 2006 tobacco settlement payment	$120.9 million

Total state revenue from tobacco excise taxes and settlement $438.8 million

Percent tobacco revenue to fund at CDC recommended level   15%

	Per Capita Recommendation
I. State and Community Interventions Multiple societal resources working together have the greatest long-term population impact.	**$4.97**
II. Health Communication Interventions Media interventions prevent tobacco use initiation, promote cessation, and shape social norms.	**$1.45**
III. Cessation Interventions Tobacco use treatment is highly cost-effective.	**$3.66**
IV. Surveillance and Evaluation Publicly financed programs should be accountable and demonstrate effectiveness.	**$1.01**
V. Administration and Management Complex, integrated programs require experienced staff to provide fiscal management, accountability, and coordination.	**$0.50**
Total	**$11.59**

Note: A justification for each program element and the rationale for the budget estimates are provided in Section A. The funding estimates presented are based on adjustments for changes in population and inflation since the 1999 publication. The recommended levels of investment (per capita and total) are presented in 2007 dollars using 2006 population estimates. These should be updated annually according to the U.S. Department of Labor Consumer Price Index and U.S. Census Bureau. The actual funding required for implementing programs will vary depending on state characteristics such as tobacco use prevalence, socio-demographic factors, and other factors. See Appendix E for data sources on deaths, costs, revenue and state-specific factors.

Office on Smoking and Health • Centers for Disease Control and Prevention
www.cdc.gov/tobacco • tobaccoinfo@cdc.gov • 1 (800) CDC INFO or 1 (800) 232-4636

CDC Recommended Annual Investment $9.0 million

Deaths in Wyoming Caused by Smoking

Annual average smoking-attributable deaths	700
Youth ages 0-17 projected to die from smoking	12,000

Annual Costs Incurred in Wyoming from Smoking

Total medical	$136 million
Medicaid medical	$37 million
Lost productivity from premature death	$155 million

State Revenue from Tobacco Excise Taxes and Settlement

FY 2006 tobacco tax revenue	$25.2 million
FY 2006 tobacco settlement payment	$14.5 million
Total state revenue from tobacco excise taxes and settlement	$39.7 million

Percent tobacco revenue to fund at CDC recommended level   23%

	Per Capita Recommendation
I. State and Community Interventions Multiple societal resources working together have the greatest long-term population impact.	$8.50
II. Health Communication Interventions Media interventions prevent tobacco use initiation, promote cessation, and shape social norms.	$2.84
III. Cessation Interventions Tobacco use treatment is highly cost-effective.	$3.77
IV. Surveillance and Evaluation Publicly financed programs should be accountable and demonstrate effectiveness.	$1.51
V. Administration and Management Complex, integrated programs require experienced staff to provide fiscal management, accountability, and coordination.	$0.76
Total	**$17.38**

Note: A justification for each program element and the rationale for the budget estimates are provided in Section A. The funding estimates presented are based on adjustments for changes in population and inflation since the 1999 publication. The recommended levels of investment (per capita and total) are presented in 2007 dollars using 2006 population estimates. These should be updated annually according to the U.S. Department of Labor Consumer Price Index and U.S. Census Bureau. The actual funding required for implementing programs will vary depending on state characteristics such as tobacco use prevalence, socio-demographic factors, and other factors. See Appendix E for data sources on deaths, costs, revenue and state-specific factors.

Office on Smoking and Health • Centers for Disease Control and Prevention
www.cdc.gov/tobacco • tobaccoinfo@cdc.gov • 1 (800) CDC INFO or 1 (800) 232-4636

Appendices

Ursula Bauer, PhD, MPH
New York State Department of Health

Tony Biglan, PhD
Oregon Research Institute

Paul G. Billings
American Lung Association

Frank J. Chaloupka, PhD
University of Illinois at Chicago

Vilma Cokkinides, PhD
American Cancer Society

Karen DeLeeuw, MSW
Colorado Department of
Public Health and Environment

Melissa Fahrenbruch, MEd
Centers for Disease Control and Prevention

Matthew C. Farrelly, PhD
RTI International

Meg Gallogly, MPH
Campaign for Tobacco-free Kids

Robert Hornik, PhD
Annenberg School for Communication

Paula Keller, MPH
University of Wisconsin School
of Medicine and Public Health

Helen Lettlow, DrPh
American Legacy Foundation

Douglas Luke, PhD
Saint Louis University School of Public Health

Judy Martin, MS
Nebraska Department of Health and Human Services

Jane Pritzl, MA

Todd Rogers, PhD
Public Health Institute

Hana Ross, PhD
American Cancer Society

Pelagie Snesrud, BSN, PHN
Centers for Disease Control and Prevention

Madeleine Solomon, MPH
American Heart Association

Colleen Stevens, MSW
California Department of Public Health

Makani Themba-Nixon
The Praxis Project

Michael Thun, MD, MS
American Cancer Society

Donna Vallone, PhD, MPH
American Legacy Foundation

Robert E. Vollinger, Jr., MSPH
National Cancer Institute

Donna Warner, MA, MBA
Massachusetts Department of Health

Funding Recommendation Formulations

In *Best Practices for Comprehensive Tobacco Control Programs—August 1999*, funding formulas were provided for the nine specific elements of a comprehensive program. These formulas were based on evidence from scientific literature and the experience of large-scale and sustained efforts of state programs in California and Massachusetts.[1]

In December 2006, technical consultation was sought from a panel of experts regarding the best available evidence to determine updated cost parameters and metrics for major components of a comprehensive tobacco control program. The panel reviewed data relevant to potential changes in the 1999 funding recommendations, including state experience and findings on program effectiveness that have emerged since the release of *Best Practices—1999*. The panel generally agreed that the published funding formulas remained sound but that technical updates were necessary.[2] A listing of participants in the expert panel is provided in Appendix A.

Funding recommendations in this publication are based on the funding formulas presented in 1999, with adjustments to specific variables to account for changes in the total population (2006), population of persons aged 18 years and older (2006), public (2006) and private (2003) school enrollment, and smoking prevalence (2006), as well as an increase to keep pace with the national cost of living (June 2007).[3-7]

The original basis for budget recommendations is as follows:[1]
- Community Programs: $850,000-$1,200,000 (statewide training and infrastructure) + $0.70-$2.00 per capita
- Tobacco-Related Disease Programs: Average of $2.8 million - $4.1 million per year
- School Programs: $500,000-$750,000 (statewide training and infrastructure) + $4-$6 per student (K-12)
- Enforcement: $150,000-$300,000 estimated range for youth access and smoke-free air enforcement + $0.43-$0.80 per capita
- Statewide Programs: $0.40-$1.00 per capita
- Counter-Marketing: $1.00-$3.00 per capita
- Cessation
  - Minimum: $1 per adult (screening) + $2 per smoker (brief counseling)
  - Maximum: $1 per adult (screening) + $2 per smoker (brief counseling) + $13.75 per smoker (50% of quitline cost for 10% of smokers) + $27.50 per smoker for NRT (assumes approximately 25% of smokers treated are covered by state-financed programs)
- Surveillance and Evaluation: 10% of program total
- Administration and Management: 5% of program total

As with the funding guidance first published in 1999, recommended annual costs can vary within the lower and upper estimates provided for each state. Therefore, to better assist

states, specific guidance is now provided regarding each state's recommended level of investment within its range. These recommended levels of annual investment factor in state-specific variables, such as the overall population; smoking prevalence; the proportion of the population uninsured or receiving publicly financed insurance or living at or near the poverty level; infrastructure costs; the number of local health units; geographic size; the targeted reach for quitline services; and the cost and complexity of conducting mass media campaigns to reach targeted audiences, such as youth, racial/ethnic minorities, or people of low socioeconomic status.[3,6,8-14]

Per capita formula adjustments for 2007 include:
- Community Programs: Upper and lower limits were adjusted for inflation. Specific state estimates within these limits took into account smoking prevalence, proportion of the population living at or below 200% of the poverty level, average wage rates for implementing public health programs, the number of local health units, and geographic size.
- Tobacco-Related Disease Programs: Total budget numbers were adjusted for inflation and distributed to each state on a per capita basis.
- School Programs: Budget numbers were adjusted for inflation and applied to state school enrollment.
- Enforcement: Budget numbers were adjusted for inflation.
- Statewide Programs: Upper and lower limits were adjusted for inflation. Specific state estimates within these limits took into account smoking prevalence, proportion of the population living at or below 200% of the poverty level, average wage rates for implementing public health programs, the number of local health units, and geographic size.
- Counter-Marketing: Upper and lower limits were adjusted for inflation. Specific state estimates within these limits took into account relative media costs and the complexity of the media market.
- Cessation:
  - Health care systems (screening and brief counseling) budget numbers were adjusted for inflation.
  - Quitline support: (number of callers enrolled in quitline) x (per person cost for counseling) + (per person cost for NRT). Formula assumes 6% of adult smokers in the state receive treatment each year.
- Surveillance and Evaluation: 10% of program total.
- Administration and Management: 5% of program total.

Multiplying state per capita funding recommendations by state population will provide the total funding recommendations presented in the total funding summary table and the state-specific pages. Because total funding recommendations are rounded to the nearest hundred thousand, the reverse calculation might produce slightly different per capita estimates. The recommended levels of investment (per capita and total) are presented in 2007 dollars using 2006 population rates. These should be updated annually according to the U.S. Department of Labor Consumer Price Index and U.S. Census Bureau.[3,7]

References

1. Centers for Disease Control and Prevention. *Best Practices for Comprehensive Tobacco Control Programs—August 1999.* Atlanta: U.S. Department of Health and Human Services; 1999.

2. Centers for Disease Control and Prevention. *Panel Review of Best Practices for Comprehensive Tobacco Control Programs.* Atlanta: U.S. Department of Health and Human Services; 2006. Available at http://www.cdc.gov/tobacco/ tobacco_control_programs/stateandcommunity/ sustainingstates/BestPracticesMeeting htm.

3. U.S. Census Bureau, Population Division. Estimates of the population by selected age groups for the United States and for Puerto Rico, July 1, 2006 (SC-EST2006-01). Release date: May 17, 2007. Available at http://www.census.gov/popest/states/ asrh/tables/SC-EST2006-01.xls.

4. National Center for Education Statistics. Digest of education statistics, 2006, Table 33: Enrollment in public elementary and secondary schools, by state or jurisdiction: fall 1990 through fall 2006. Available at http://nces.ed.gov/programs/digest/d06/ tables/dt06_033.asp.

5. National Center for Education Statistics. Digest of education statistics, 2006, Table 59: Private elementary and secondary schools, enrollment, teachers, and high school graduates, by state: selected years, 1997 through 2003. Available at http://nces.ed.gov/programs/digest/d06/ tables/dt06_059.asp.

6. Centers for Disease Control and Prevention. Behavioral Risk Factor Surveillance System, Prevalence Data: Tobacco Use – 2006. Available at http://apps.nccd.cdc.gov/brfss/list.asp?cat=TU&yr=2 006&qkey=4396&state=UB.

7. U.S. Department of Labor, Bureau of Labor Statistics. Consumer Price Index. Available at http://data.bls.gov/cgi-bin/surveymost?cu.

8. U.S. Census Bureau. Current Population Survey Annual Social and Economic Supplement, March 2006. Available at http://www.census.gov/hhes/ www/cpstc/cps_table_creator html.

9. U.S. Census Bureau. Current Population Survey Annual Social and Economic Supplement, March 2006. Available at http://www.census.gov/hhes/ www/cpstc/cps_table_creator html.

10. U.S. Census Bureau. Current Population Survey Annual Social and Economic Supplement, March 2006. Available at http://pubdb3.census.gov/ macro/032006/pov/new46_000.htm.

11. U.S. Department of Labor, Bureau of Labor Statistics. Quarterly Census of Employment and Wages, Administration of Public Health Programs, August 9, 2007. Available at http://data.bls.gov/ cgi-bin/dsrv?en.

12. National Association of County and City Health Officials. Local health units, by state. Personal communication, July 17, 2007.

13. U.S. Census Bureau, American FactFinder. Geographic Comparison Table: Population, Housing Units, and Density: 2000. Available at http://factfinder.census.gov/servlet/GCTTable?_ bm=y&-ds_name=DEC_2000_SF1_U&- CONTEXT=gct&-mt_name=DEC_2000_ SF1_U_GCTPH1_US9&-redoLog=false&- _caller=geoselect&-geo_id=&-format=US-9|US- 9S&-_lang=en.

14. Nielsen Media Research, 2006 Spot television cost estimates per state.Unpublished data, 2006.

Program and Policy Recommendations for Comprehensive Tobacco Control Programs

Guide to Community Preventive Services Tobacco Control Recommendations[1]

Excerpt from Task Force on Community Preventive Services' *The Guide to Community Preventive Services: What Works to Promote Health?*

"Based on the evidence of effectiveness documented in the scientific literature, recommendations from the Task Force support the following population-based tobacco prevention and control efforts:

- Clean indoor air legislation prohibiting tobacco use in indoor public and private workplaces.
- Federal, state, and local efforts to increase tobacco product excise taxes as an effective public health intervention to promote tobacco use cessation and to reduce the initiation of tobacco use among youth.
- The funding and implementation of long-term, high-intensity mass media campaigns using paid broadcast times and media messages developed through formative research.
- Proactive telephone cessation support services (quit lines).
- Reduced or eliminated co-payments for effective cessation therapies.
- Reminder systems for healthcare providers.
- Combinations of efforts to mobilize communities to identify and reduce the commercial availability of tobacco products to youth.

"In reflecting the available evidence on effectiveness, recommendations from the Task Force confirm the importance of coordinated or combined intervention efforts in tobacco prevention. Evidence of effectiveness in efforts to reduce tobacco use among youth through access restrictions, to disseminate anti-tobacco messages through mass media, and to assist tobacco users in their efforts to quit via telephone comes predominantly from the studies that implemented these interventions in combination with other strategies."

Healthy People 2010 Policy Goals[2,3]

Selected national health objectives addressing policy interventions to reduce tobacco use:

27-8   Increase insurance coverage of evidence-based treatment for nicotine dependency among managed care organizations to 100% and among Medicaid programs to all 50 states and the District of Columbia.

27-9   Reduce the proportion of children who are regularly exposed to tobacco smoke at home to 6%.

27-10   Reduce the proportion of nonsmokers exposed to environmental tobacco smoke to 63%.

27-11   Increase smoke-free and tobacco-free environments in schools, including all school facilities, property, vehicles, and school events to 100%.

27-12   Increase the proportion of persons covered by indoor worksite policies that prohibit smoking to 100%.

27-13   Establish laws on smoke-free indoor air that prohibit smoking in public places and worksites (including private and public worksites, restaurants, public transportation, day care centers, retail stores, and bars) in all 50 states and the District of Columbia.

27-14   Reduce the illegal sales rate to minors through enforcement of laws prohibiting the sale of tobacco products to minors to all 50 states and the District of Columbia.

27-15   Increase the number of states (including the District of Columbia) that suspend or revoke state retail licenses for violations of laws prohibiting the sale of tobacco to minors to 51.

27-16   Reduce the proportion of adolescents and young adults who are exposed to tobacco advertising and promotion to 67% for magazines and newspaper and to 25% for Internet.

27-19   Eliminate laws that preempt stronger tobacco control laws in all 50 states and the District of Columbia.

27-21   Increase the average federal and state tax on cigarettes to $2.00 and expand the number of states (and the District of Columbia) with higher smokeless tobacco taxes over the decade to 51.

References

1. Zaza S, Briss PA, Harris KW, editors. *The Guide to Community Preventive Services: What Works to Promote Health?* New York: Oxford University Press; 2005.

2. U.S. Department of Health and Human Services. *Healthy People 2010, Volume 2.* Washington, DC: U.S. Government Printing Office; 2000.

3. U.S. Department of Health and Human Services. *Healthy People 2010, Midcourse Review.* Washington, DC: U.S. Government Printing Office; 2006.

Because some populations within the United States experience a disproportionate health and economic burden from tobacco use, a focus on reducing tobacco-related disparities is necessary. Identifying and eliminating tobacco-related disparities is a primary goal of every state tobacco control program, along with preventing initiation of tobacco use, promoting tobacco cessation, and eliminating exposure to secondhand smoke.

Tobacco-related disparities are "differences in patterns, prevention, and treatment of tobacco use; the risk, incidence, morbidity, mortality, and burden of tobacco-related illness that exist among specific population groups in the United States; and related differences in capacity and infrastructure, access to resources, and environmental tobacco smoke exposure."[1] Measuring these kinds of characteristics in a population assessment will identify the high-risk populations within a state or community.

Focusing efforts on the identification and elimination of tobacco-related disparities may close the gaps in prevalence of tobacco use and access to effective treatment, thus alleviating the disproportionate health and economic burden experienced by some sectors of the population. These subgroups may be distinguished, for example, by factors such as race or ethnicity, age, socioeconomic status, geographic location, mental health, sexual orientation, level of education or acculturation, and they may differ from state to state.

State tobacco control programs collaborate with stakeholders to build capacity and infrastructure. This strategy is useful in guiding the public health system in developing policies and practices that reflect the principles of inclusion and cultural competency. In addition, clear leadership and dedicated resources are essential to develop and implement a strong strategic plan and develop tobacco control efforts devoted to identifying and eliminating tobacco-related disparities. Reaching the national goal of eliminating health disparities related to tobacco use will necessitate improved collection and use of standardized data to correctly identify disparities in tobacco use, health outcomes, and efficacy of prevention programs among various population groups.[2] The use of oversampling, combining multiple years of data, and qualitative methods are often necessary to reflect changes in knowledge, attitudes, and behaviors in specific population groups.

This guidance is based on information about state practices, published scientific findings, and input from external partners. This guidance highlights the presumed minimum infrastructure and capacity needed by state and territorial tobacco control programs to pursue strategic activities that would identify and eliminate tobacco-related disparities.[3]

Activities to support reaching this goal may include:
- Conducting a population assessment to guide efforts
- Identifying and assembling a diverse and inclusive stakeholder group
- Prioritizing reduction in tobacco-related disparities and assessing capacity
- Developing a strategic plan
- Funding community organizations to implement proven or promising interventions
- Providing culturally competent technical assistance and training to grantees and partners
- Evaluating intervention efficacy and refining efforts

Initiatives for the strategic plan may include the following activities:

- Eliminating gaps in the data for identifying populations experiencing tobacco-related disparities
- Creating partnerships to maximize resources and reach of interventions
- Integrating efforts to eliminate disparities throughout all tobacco prevention and control activities
- Developing culturally competent materials and approaches
- Educating partners and decision makers about pro-tobacco influences and the disproportionate tobacco burden affecting identified populations
- Passing smoke-free policies in all worksites and public places
- Increasing the unit price of tobacco products
- Eliminating preemption from statewide tobacco control laws
- Securing funding to sustain data collection and intervention efforts
- Expanding and tailoring quitline services to serve diverse populations
- Identifying culturally competent communication interventions
- Obtaining comprehensive Medicaid coverage of tobacco use treatments

Core Resources

Starr G, Rogers T, Schooley M, Porter S, Wiesen E, Jamison N. *Key Outcome Indicators for Evaluating Comprehensive Tobacco Control Programs.* Atlanta: Centers for Disease Control and Prevention; 2005. Available at: http://www.cdc.gov/tobacco/tobacco_control_programs/surveillance_evaluation/key_outcome/index.htm.

MacDonald G, Starr G, Schooley M, Yee SL, Klimowski K, Turner K. *Introduction to Program Evaluation for Comprehensive Tobacco Control Programs.* Atlanta: Centers for Disease Control and Prevention; 2001. Available at http://www.cdc.gov/tobacco/tobacco_control_programs/surveillance_evaluation/evaluation_manual/index htm.

U.S. Department of Health and Human Services. *Tobacco Use Among U.S. Racial/Ethnic Minority Groups—African Americans, American Indians and Alaska Natives, Asian Americans and Pacific Islanders, and Hispanics: A Report of the Surgeon General.* Atlanta: U.S. Department of Health and Human Services, Centers for Disease Control and Prevention, National Center for Chronic Disease Prevention and Health Promotion, Office on Smoking and Health; 1998. Available at http://www.cdc.gov/tobacco/data_statistics/sgr/sgr_1998/index htm.

U.S. Department of Health and Human Services. *Reducing Tobacco Use: A Report of the Surgeon General.* Atlanta: U.S. Department of Health and Human Services, Centers for Disease Control and Prevention, National Center for Chronic Disease Prevention and Health Promotion, Office on Smoking and Health; 2000. Available at http://www.cdc.gov/tobacco/data_statistics/sgr/sgr_2000/index htm.

References

1. Fagan P, King G, Lawrence D, Petrucci SA, Robinson RG, Banks D, et al. Eliminating tobacco-related health disparities: directions for future research. *American Journal of Public Health* 2004;94:211–217.

2. U.S. Department of Health and Human Services. *Reducing Tobacco Use: A Report of the Surgeon General.* Atlanta: US Department of Health and Human Services, Centers for Disease Control and Prevention, National Center for Chronic Disease Prevention and Health Promotion, Office on Smoking and Health; 2000.

3. Starr G, Rogers T, Schooley M, Porter S, Wiesen E, Jamison N. *Key Outcome Indicators for Evaluating Comprehensive Tobacco Control Programs.* Atlanta: Centers for Disease Control and Prevention; 2005.

Deaths Caused by Smoking

Annual average smoking-attributable deaths:
- Source of data: Smoking-Attributable Mortality, Morbidity, and Economic Costs (SAMMEC). Available at http://apps.nccd.cdc.gov/sammec/. (Login required.)
- Data are annual averages among adults aged 35 years and older, from 1997–2001. These estimates do not include deaths related to burns or secondhand smoke.
- Smoking-attributable death totals are rounded to the nearest hundred.

Youth projected to die from smoking:
- Source of initial data: Smoking-Attributable Mortality, Morbidity, and Economic Costs (SAMMEC). Available at http://apps.nccd.cdc.gov/sammec/. (Login required.)
- This measure is calculated from estimates of youth projected to start smoking as well as estimates of premature deaths attributable to smoking among continuing smokers and among those who quit after 35 years of age.
- The following source provides a more complete description of the methodology: Centers for Disease Control and Prevention. Projected Smoking-Related Deaths Among Youth—United States. *MMWR* 1996;(45)44:977–984.
- Youth projected to start smoking: The average prevalence of smoking among adults aged 18–30 years for each state from the 2003–2004 BRFSS was used to estimate the future prevalence of smoking during early adulthood for the birth cohorts currently aged 0–17 years. The number of people aged 0–17 years in each state was obtained from U.S. Census Bureau data (July 1, 2004 estimates). Hawaii completed 3 of 12 months of interviews in 2004; these data are not available in the aggregate 2004 dataset.
- Figures are rounded to the nearest thousand.

Annual Cost from Smoking

Total medical:
- Source of data: Centers for Disease Control and Prevention. Sustaining State Programs for Tobacco Control: Data Highlights 2006. Atlanta: Centers for Disease Control and Prevention, National Center for Chronic Disease Prevention and Health Promotion, Office on Smoking and Health; 2006. Available at http://www.cdc.gov/tobacco/data_statistics/state_data/data_highlights/2006/index.htm.
- Total figures are rounded to the nearest million.

Medicaid medical only:
- Source of data: Centers for Disease Control and Prevention. *Sustaining State Programs for Tobacco Control: Data Highlights 2006.* Atlanta: Centers for Disease Control and Prevention, National Center for Chronic Disease Prevention and Health Promotion, Office on Smoking and Health; 2006. Available at http://www.cdc.gov/tobacco/data_statistics/state_data/data_highlights/2006/index.htm.
- Total figures are rounded to the nearest million.

Lost productivity:
- Source of data: Centers for Disease Control and Prevention. *Sustaining State Programs for Tobacco Control: Data Highlights 2006.* Atlanta: Centers for Disease Control and Prevention, National Center for Chronic Disease Prevention and Health Promotion, Office on Smoking and Health; 2006. Available at http://www.cdc.gov/tobacco/data_statistics/state_data/data_highlights/2006/index.htm.
- Total figures are rounded to the nearest million.

State Revenue from Tobacco Excise Taxes and Settlement

Tobacco product tax revenue
- Source of data: Orzechowski W, Walker RC. *The Tax Burden on Tobacco: Historical Compilation, 2006.* Tables 9 and 12. Arlington, VA: Orzechowski and Walker; 2006.
- Total figures are rounded to the nearest hundred thousand.

Tobacco settlement payment in 2006
- Source of data: Centers for Disease Control and Prevention. State Tobacco Activities Tracking and Evaluation (STATE) System. Available at http://apps.nccd.cdc.gov/statesystem/.
- Data were provided for the STATE System by the National Association of Attorneys General for 46 states and District of Columbia that participated in the Master Settlement Agreement (MSA). Payments for four non-MSA states were obtained by direct contact with those states.
- Total figures are rounded to the nearest hundred thousand.

Data Sources Used in Funding Recommendation Formulas

Overall population by age
- Source of data: U.S. Census Bureau, Population Division. Estimates of the population by selected age groups for the United States and for Puerto Rico, July 1, 2006 (SC-EST2006-01). Release date: May 17, 2007. Available at http://www. census.gov/popest/states/asrh/tables/SC-EST2006-01.xls.

Smoking prevalence
- Source of data: Centers for Disease Control and Prevention. Behavioral Risk Factor Surveillance System, Prevalence Data: Tobacco Use – 2006. Available at http://apps.nccd.cdc.gov/brfss/list.asp?cat=TU&yr=2006&qkey=4396&state=UB.

Proportion of adult civilian population with health insurance coverage
- Source of data: U.S. Census Bureau. Current Population Survey Annual Social and Economic Supplement, March 2006. Available at http://www.census.gov/hhes/www/cpstc/cps_table_creator.html. (To access data, select: 2006, Adult Civilian Persons, Row: States, Column: Health Insurance Coverage, Percentages by: Health Insurance Coverage.)

Proportion of adult civilian population receiving Medicaid
- Source of data: U.S. Census Bureau. Current Population Survey Annual Social and Economic Supplement, March 2006. Available at http://www.census.gov/hhes/www/cpstc/cps_table_creator.html. (To access data, select: 2006, Adult Civilian Persons, Row: States, Column: Health Insurance: Medicaid, Percentages by: Health Insurance: Medicaid)

Living at or below 200% of poverty level
- Source of data: U.S. Census Bureau. Current Population Survey Annual Social and Economic Supplement, March 2006. Available at http://pubdb3.census.gov/macro/032006/pov/new46_000.htm.

Cost of average annual salary to implement public health programs
- Source of data: U.S. Department of Labor, Bureau of Labor Statistics. Quarterly Census of Employment and Wages, Administration of Public Health Programs, August 9, 2007. Available at http://data.bls.gov/cgi-bin/dsrv?en. (To access data, <Control> select: 10, 92, 923, 9231, and 92312, <Next Form>; using Search Area, enter "??000" in Code box to select all, <Search>; highlight and select list of all states, <Next Form>; select 2, <Next Form>; 5, <Next Form>; 0, <Next Form>; years 2005-2007 and Format 1 <Retrieve Data>)

Data Sources

Number of local health units
- Source of data: National Association of County and City Health Officials. Local health units, by state. Unpublished data, 2007.

Geographic size
- Source of data: U.S. Census Bureau, American FactFinder. Geographic Comparison Table: Population, Housing Units, and Density: 2000. Available at http://factfinder.census.gov/servlet/GCTTable?_bm=y&-ds_name=DEC_2000_SF1_U&-CONTEXT=gct&-mt_name=DEC_2000_SF1_U_GCTPH1_US9&-redoLog=false&-_caller=geoselect&-geo_id=&-format=US-9|US-9S&-_lang=en.

Designated market area cost and reach of targeted audience
- Source of data: Nielsen Media Research, 2006 Spot Television Cost Estimates per State. Unpublished data, 2006.

Private school K-12 enrollment
- Source of data: National Center for Education Statistics. Digest of education statistics, 2006, Table 33: Enrollment in public elementary and secondary schools, by state or jurisdiction: fall 1990 through fall 2006. Available at http://nces.ed.gov/programs/digest/d06/tables/dt06_033.asp.

Public school K-12 enrollment
- Source of data: National Center for Education Statistics. Digest of education statistics, 2006, Table 59: Private elementary and secondary schools, enrollment, teachers, and high school graduates, by state: selected years, 1997 through 2003. Available at http://nces.ed.gov/programs/digest/d06/tables/dt06_059.asp.

Rate of inflation
- Source of data: U.S. Department of Labor, Bureau of Labor Statistics. Consumer Price Index. Available at http://data.bls.gov/cgi-bin/surveymost?cu. (To access data, select U.S. All items, 1982-84=100 - CUUR0000SA0. Base is annual 1997 index.)

www.ingramcontent.com/pod-product-compliance
Lightning Source LLC
Chambersburg PA
CBHW080301180526
45167CB00006B/2620